POISON DAMSELS: TOXIC RIDDLES FOR TOXIC DETECTIVE

An Indian Society of Toxicology Initiative

Dr Vivekanshu Verma
Dr Vijay Vasudev Pillay
Dr Shiv Rattan Kochar
Dr Prateek Rastogi
Dr Vatsal Panwar

© Indian Society of Toxicology

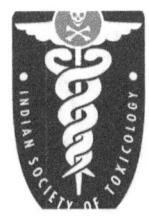

ISBN: 9798695341379

Cover design by: Mr Vishwendra Verma, B. Tech, MBA

Library of Indian Society of Toxicology Archives Number: 2018675309

Printed in the Poison Control Centre
Amrita Institute of Medical Science,
Ponekkara, P. O, Kochi, Kerala - 682041.

CONTENTS

Poison Damsels: Toxic Riddles for the Toxic Detectives

Vivekanshu Verma
Vijay Vasudev Pillay
Shiv Rattan Kochar
Prateek Rastogi
Vatsal Panwar

An Indian Society of Toxicology Initiative

An Indian Society of Toxicology Initiative

For Crime Scene Investigators (CSi), Toxicologists, Police Officers, CID, CBI officers, Lawyers, Judges, Magistrates, Legal counsels, Students, Forensic Scientists, Doctors, Toxicology Nurses & Emergency Paramedics

Dr Vivekanshu Verma, MBBS, Postgraduate Diploma in Forensic Medicine & Toxicology, Fellow of Indian Society of Toxicology, Associate consultant, Emergency & Trauma care, Medanta-The Medicity, Gurugram, Honorary Toxicology Expert, Central Bureau of Investigation

Dr Vijay Vasudev Pillay, MBBS, MD Forensic Medicine & Toxicology, Chief, Poison Control Centre, Professor & Head, Forensic Medicine & Toxicology, Amrita School of Medicine, Amrita Vishwa Vidyapeetham, Cochin, Kerala

Dr Shiv Rattan Kochar, MBBS, MD Forensic Medicine & Toxicology, Senior Professor, Forensic Medicine. Chief Vigilance Officer, Metro MANAS Arogya Sadan Heart Care & Multispecialty Hospital, Directorate of Medical Education, Jaipur (Rajasthan)

Dr Prateek Rastogi, MBBS, MD, PGDMLE, PGDCFS, PGCMNCPA, PGCTM, Dip. Cyber Law, FAGE, FAIMER Fellow (MUFILIPE-Manipal), Former President, Indian Society of Toxicology(2018-19), Professor, Department of Forensic Medicine & Toxicology, Kasturba Medical College, Mangalore, Karnataka

Dr Vatsal Panwar, BAMS, PGC Panchakarma, PGD Clinical Cosmetology, Aesthetic Consultant, Delhi-NCR

VISH / WISH

Our Indian toxicologists wish to know,

How the term Vish (विष) was coined?

Wish & Vish=विष (are homophonic sound-alike, wish is English word, and vish is Sanskrit word, but contradictory meaning)

संस्कृत में विष् धातु में कृ प्रत्यय लगकर विष संज्ञा बनी है, जिसका अर्थ है प्रसरणशील = जो शरीर में जाकर एकदम फैल जाऐ, और शारीरिक एवं मानसिक विषाद उत्पन्न करे ॥

उत्तरोत्तर धातु में जल्दी से फैलने के कारण विष संज्ञा बनी है ॥

विषाक्त = Toxicity

सुश्रुत संहिता defined Toxicology termed as अगदतन्त्रं :

सर्पकीटलूतामूषिकादिदष्टविषव्यंजनार्थं विविधविषसंयोगोपशमनार्थं च ।

Explanation:

सर्प, कीड़े, मकड़ी, चूहे के काटने से उत्पन्न विष लक्षणों की पहचान तथा अनेक प्रकार के स्वाभाविक कृत्रिम और संयोग विषों से उत्पन्न विकारों के प्रशमन का वर्णन जहाँ हो उसे अगदतंत्र कहते हैं ॥

Rat-bites do transmit rabies & tetanus (fatal illnesses), causing deaths in past, so considered toxic in this definition.

विषकन्या

रिपवो विक्रमाक्रान्ता ये च स्वे कृत्यतां गताः।

सिसृक्षवः क्रोधविषं विवरं प्राप्य तद्दृशम्।।

विषैर्निहन्युर्निपुणं नृपतिं दुष्टचेतसः।

स्त्रियो वा विविधान् योगान् कदाचित्सुभगेच्छया।।

विषकन्योपयोगाद्धा क्षणाज्जह्यादसुन्नरः।

तस्माद्वैद्येन सततं विषाद्रक्ष्यो नराधिपः।।

- (सुश्रुत संहिता कल्पस्थान अ० १)

In ancient times the King was supposed to be the most important person of the state and saving his precious life was considered as the most essential task, for his ministers specially the Raj Vaidya or Chief Physician.

In the above shloka, Acharya Sushrut explains that, enemies who were conquered & defeated by the King with bravery and courage, might approach King's own servants and relatives having personal venegance, may conspire against the King, and to take revenge , concoct poisonous compounds and give the same to him.

Powerful though the King may be, but the enemies take advantage of his weak points (like attraction to beautiful women, and alcohol) and are constantly looking for the chance to accomplish their task in killing the King.

Acharya Sushrut also explains that sometimes ladies are found to administer the person(husband or lover) with various preparations (food and drinks) which have poison in them.

They do this in order to secure their affection and good luck.

And sometimes it is found that by embracing a Vishkanya (girl who acts as poison) kills the person instantly.

Hence it is imperative duty of the chief physician to guard the king from the conspirators who try to poison him.

The above shloka is further elaborated by Acharya Dalhana who was the commentator of sushruta samhita

He says that the girl or Vishkanya who is a sent to the king can kill the him with her embracing touch , perspiration and by sexual intercourse.

हन्ति स्पृशन्तौ स्वेदेन , गम्यमाना च मैथुने।

पक्वं वृन्तादिव फलं प्रशातयति मेहनम्।।

(निबंधसंग्रह)

Acharya Vaghbhatt has also mentioned Vishkanya in Ashtang Samgrah

न च कन्यामविदितां संस्पृशेदपरीक्षिताम्।

विविधान् कुर्वते योगान् कुशला: खलुमानवा:।

आजन्मविषसंयोगात् कन्या विषमयी कृता।।

स्पृशोच्छवासादिभिर्हन्ति तस्यास्यत्वेतत् परीक्षणम्।

तद्धस्तकेशसंस्पृशार्न् म्लायते पुष्पपल्लवौ।।

शय्यायां मुत्कुणैर्वस्त्रे यूकाभि: स्नानवारिणा।

जन्तुभिर्म्रियते ज्ञात्वा तामेवं दूरतस्त्यजेत्।

(अष्टांग संग्रह सूत्रस्थान अ० ८)

In the above shloka explains how to protect the King from enemies and conspirators who can poison him by trying various methods. Therefore it was advisable for the king to not touch or embrace a woman who is a complete stranger , a woman whose family background is not known or whose conduct and behaviour is mysterious or a woman who has not been examined by the chief physician.

Right from the time of birth girl was administered with poison so that her body contains considerable amount of poison. The girl with the poison in her body generally killed the person with her touch and exhaled breath.

To ascertain whether the girl has poison in her body following methods were used by the chief physician. If flowers, leaves and fruits gets shrivel with

The touch of her hand and hair, if bugs don't survive in her bedding, if insects and animals get killed by consuming water which the girl has used for bathing then this kind of girl should be strictly avoided by the king.

To transform a girl into Vishkanya, she was given poison in a small quantity right from the time of birth and the dose of poison was slowly and gradually increased over the period time until her entire body, breath and secretions become poisonous . Some ancient texts mention that the girl was never fed salt in the diet if she has to turn into a Vishkanya.

If a person has sexual intercourse with such a girl he dies a dreadful death. Woman with communicable sexual disease is also considered as Vishkanya.

The use of Vishkanya is mentioned in an ancient play by Vishakhdutta in his play named Mudrarakshas written in 8th century where Chanakya the famous Indian economist and minister of King chandragupta failed the plan of Dhananand to kill The King Chandragupta Maurya, but Chanakya diverted her to kill Pravartak.

कन्यां तीव्रविषप्रोगविषमां कृत्वा

POISON MAIDEN:

विष-कन्या

Poison Damsels have been described as Biological Weapons in ancient warfare & its Pharmacogenomics

Many cases of lethal intoxication had been reported from antiquity.

We get the reference of Vishkanya, food poisoning and many other types of poisoning in **Sushruta Samhita**, **Ashtanga Hridaya**, and **Arthashastra** of Kautilya.

The remedies to these poisons, methods to identify poisonous foods, drinks, oils, etc., are also mentioned in this text.

Roy, Kaushik India's Historic Battles: From Alexander the Great to Kargil. Orient Blackswan. 2004. p. 24. ISBN 9788178241098.

अगदतंत्र

(Agada Tantra)

Agada means antidote drug and tantra means a system to heal the body.

The science of the treatment of poisons is Agada Tantra and it was the ancient sanskrit name of **Toxicology.**

The treatment of diseases caused by the bite of poisonous creatures comes under the branch of science, damstra.

In olden days, this branch of medical science was well developed and there were expert physicians who used to treat only cases of poisoning.

In Arthashastra of Kautilya, they are named as jangalavid.

In Kadambari (कादंबरी) novel of Banabhatta, they were named **jangulika.**

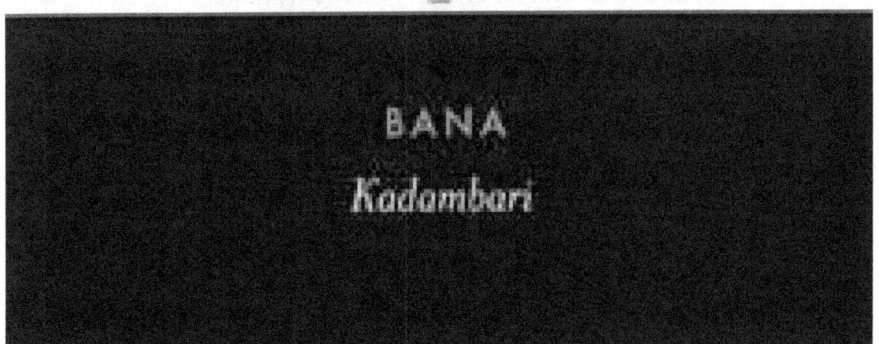

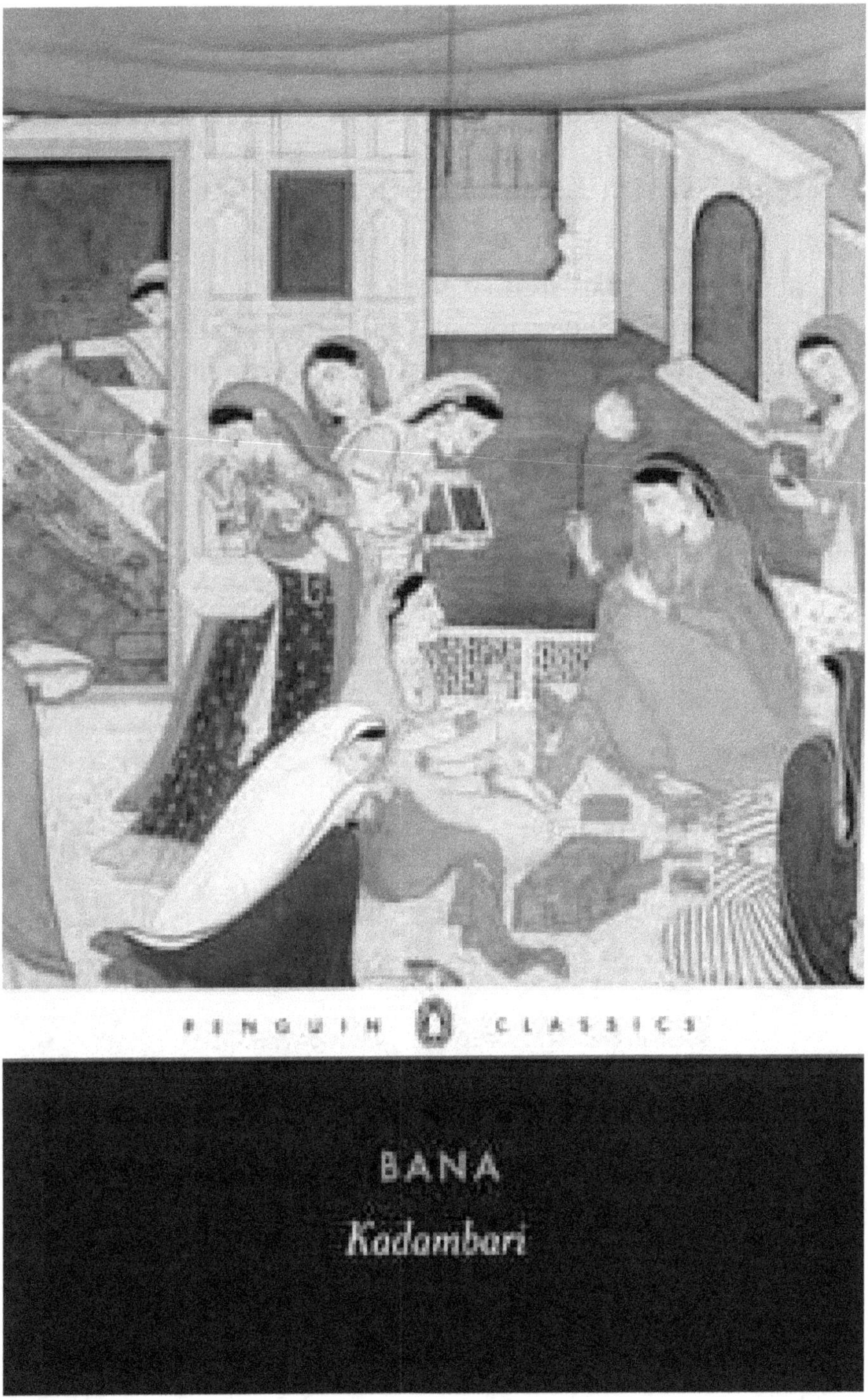

PENGUIN CLASSICS

BANA

Kadambari

Kadambari is a lyrical prose romance that narrates the love story of Kadambari, a Gandharva princess, and Chandrapida, a prince who is eventually revealed to be the moon god.

Acclaimed as a great literary work, it is replete with eloquent descriptions of palaces, forests, mountains, gardens, sunrises and sunsets and love in separation and fulfillment.

Featuring an intriguing parrot-narrator, the story progresses as a delightful romantic thriller played out in the magical realms between this world and the other, in which the earthly and the divine blend in idyllic splendour.

https://tableforchange.com/agada-tantra-study-of-poisons-in-ayurveda/

तंत्र-मंत्र-यंत्र

(तन- मन)

Tantra (तंत्र) heals body (Tan =तन = Body)

Mantra (मंत्र) heals the mindful soul (मन)

Yantra is Scientific Technology (यान)

Aeroplane = वायु यान

Dr. Devdutt Pattnaik (Doctor, Mythologist & Scholar) explains nicely on attitude (mantra), skills (tantra) and technology (yantra).

Traditionally, Vedic technologies were classified into three: the mantra (that works on the 'mana' or mind), the tantra (that works on the 'tana' or body), and the yantra (that technology or instrument that is independent of the mind or body).

Mantras sought to create conceptual clarity or emotional stability. Tantras were behaviors (chanting, fasting, celibacy, pilgrimages, postures, breath control) that used the body to solve problems, without placing any demand on the head or heart.

And finally there were the yantras (idols, images, and geometrical patterns) located outside humans, designed to impact the world around us without putting any pressure on the mind or body.

Yantras were about plug & play: just wear the talisman and see fortune turn.

AYURVEDA & विषकन्या

रिपवो विक्रमाक्रान्ता ये च स्वे कृत्यतां गता:।

सिसृक्षव: क्रोधविषं विवरं प्राप्य तदृशम्।।

विषैर्निहन्युर्निपुणं नृपतिं दुष्टचेतस:।

स्त्रियो वा विविधान् योगान् कदाचित्सुभगेच्छया।।

विषकन्योपयोगाद्वा क्षणाज्जह्यादसुनर:।

तस्माद्वैद्येन सततं विषाद्रक्ष्यो नराधिप:।।

(**सुश्रुत** संहिता कल्पस्थान अ० १)

Sloka Explained:

In ancient times the King was supposed to be the most important person of the state and saving his precious life was considered was the most essential task for his ministers specially the Raj-Vaidya or Chief Physician to the king.

In the above shloka Acharya **Sushrut** explains that enemies who are conquered with bravery and courage and King's own servants and relatives sometimes in fit of anger and to take revenge , concoct poisonous compounds and the same to him, powerful though he may be , but the enemies take advantage of any weak point and because they are constantly looking for the chance to accomplish their task in killing the King.

Acharya **Sushrut** also explains that sometimes ladies are found to administer the person(husband or lover) with various preparations (food and drinks) which have poison in them.

They do this in order to secure their affection and good luck.

And sometimes it is found that by embracing a Vishkanya (girl who acts as poison) kills the person instantly.

Hence it is imperative duty of the chief physician to guard the king from against the conspirators who try to poison him.

The above shloka is further elaborated by Acharya Dalhana who was the commentator of sushruta samhita.

He says that the girl or Vishkanya who is a sent to the king can kill the him with her embracing touch , perspiration and by sexual intercourse.

TIPS TO AVOID VISHKANYA

न च कन्यामविदितां संस्पृशेदपरीक्षिताम्।

विविधान् कुर्वते योगान् कुशला: खलुमानवा:।

आजन्मविषसंयोगात् कन्या विषमयी कृता।।

स्पृशोच्छवासादिभिर्हन्ति तस्यास्त्वेतत् परीक्षणम्।

तद्धस्तकेशसंस्पृशार्न् म्लायते पुष्पपल्लवौ।।

शय्यायां मुत्कुणैर्वस्त्रे यूकाभि: स्नानवारिणा।

जन्तुभिर्म्रियते ज्ञात्वा तामेवं दूरतस्त्यजेत्।

(अष्टांग संग्रह सूत्रस्थान अ० ८)

Acharya Vaghbhatt has also mentioned Vishkanya in Ashtang Samgrah:

In the above shloka, protection of the Ruler or King from enemies and conspirators who can to poison him trying various methods.

Therefore it was advisable for the king to not touch a woman who is a complete stranger, a woman whose family background is not known or whose conduct and behaviour is unknown or a woman who has not been examined by the chief physician.

Right from the time of birth, girl was administered with poison so that her body contains considerable amount of poison.

The girl with the poison in her body generally killed the person with her touch and exhaled breath.

To ascertain whether the girl has poison in her body following methods were used by the chief physician.:-

If flowers, leaves and fruits gets shrivel with touch of her hand and hair, if bugs don't survive in her bedding, if insects and animals get killed by consuming water which the girl has used for bathing then this kind of girl should be strictly avoided or never let her go near to the king.

To transform a girl into Vishkanya, she was given poison in a small quantity right from the time of birth and the dose of poison was slowly and gradually increased over the period time until her entire body, breath and secretions become poisonous.

If a person has sexual intercourse with such a girl he dies a dreadful death.

Woman with communicable sexual disease was also considered as Vishkanya.

CHANAKYA & VISHKANYA

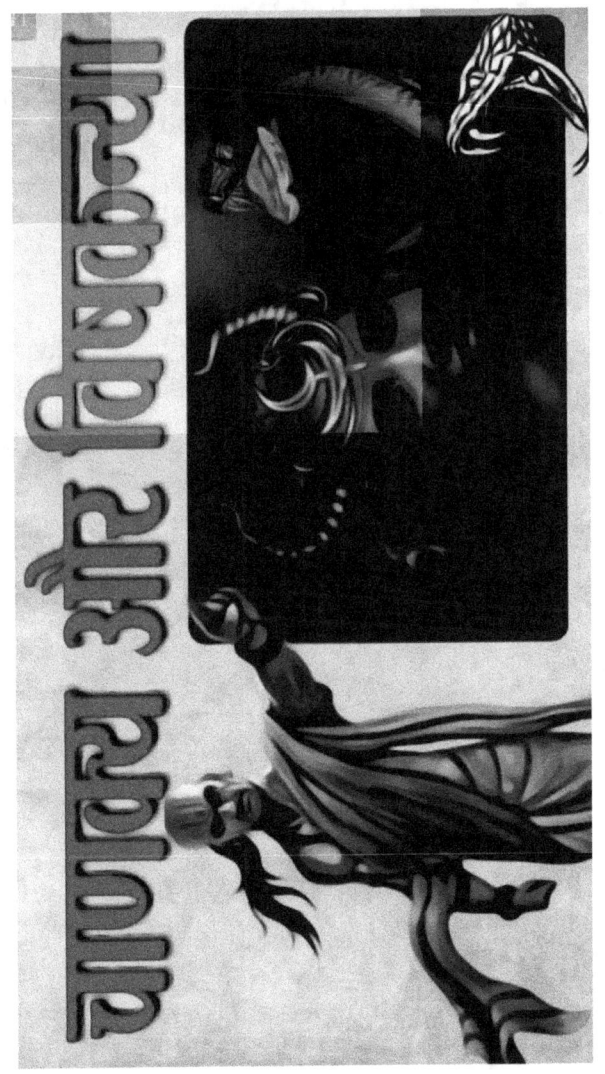

SKILL TO KILL

Poison Damsel's blood and bodily fluids were purportedly poisonous to other humans, as was mentioned in the ancient Indian treatise on statecraft, Arthashastra, written by **Acharya Kautilya**, the Chanakya, an adviser and a prime minister to the first Maurya Emperor Chandragupta (c. 340–293 BCE).

He was skilled in he art of toxicology, not just to kill, but had the skill to heal, as he was expert in medicine, law & science.

Two books are attributed to Chanakya: Arthashastra, and Chanakya Niti, also known as Chanakya Neeti-shastra.

Chanakya Niti is a collection of aphorisms, said to be selected by Chanakya from the various shastras.[

The Arthashastra identifies its author as Kauṭilya, a clan name, except for one verse that refers to him by the personal name of Vishnugupta.

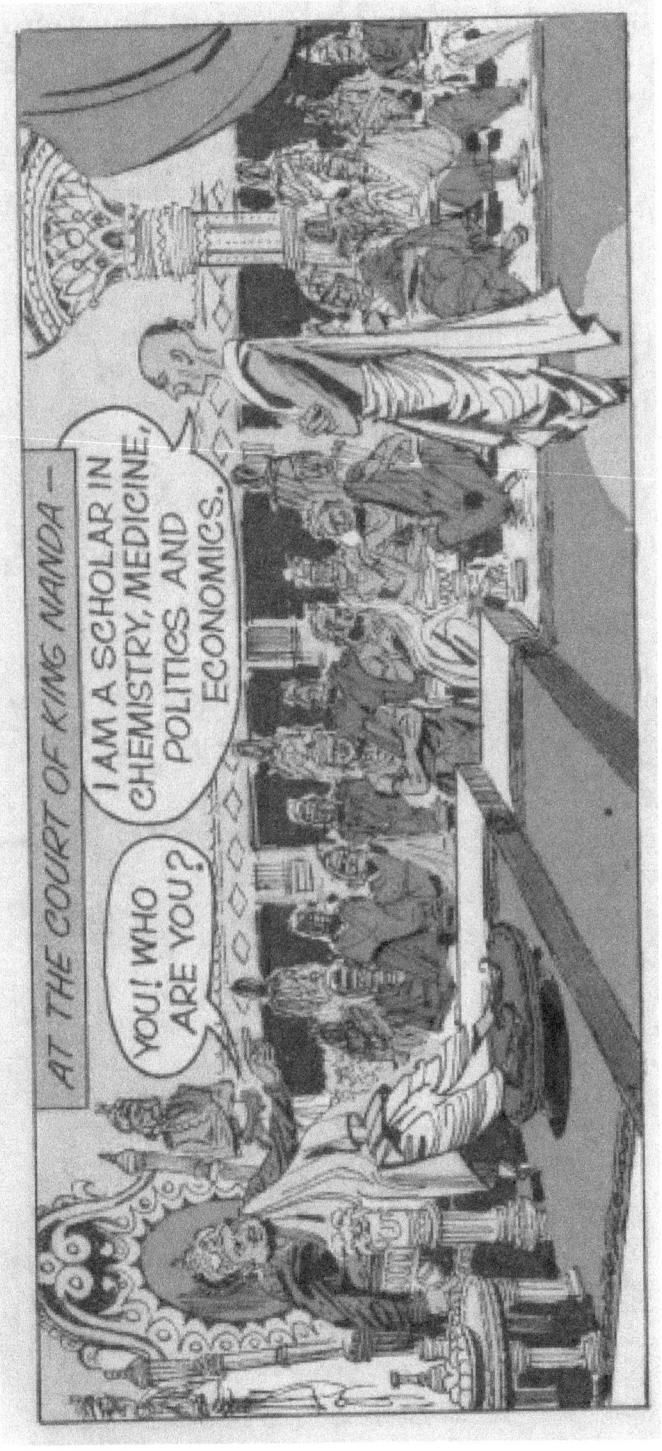

According to the Buddhist text Mahabodhivamsa, Dhana Nanda (died c. 321 BCE) was the last ruler of the Nanda dynasty in Ancient India.

He was the youngest of the eight brothers of the dynasty's founder Ugrasena (also known as Mahapadma Nanda).

Chanakya, a Brahmin who was insulted by him, vowed to overthrow him, and raised an army that invaded the Nanda capital Pataliputra and **killed** him.

Chanakya then installed his own protege Chandragupta Maurya on the throne.

Chaurasia, RS. History of ancient India: earliest times to 1000 A.D. Atlantic Publishers & Dist. (1 January 2002). p. 100. ISBN 978-81-269-0027-5.

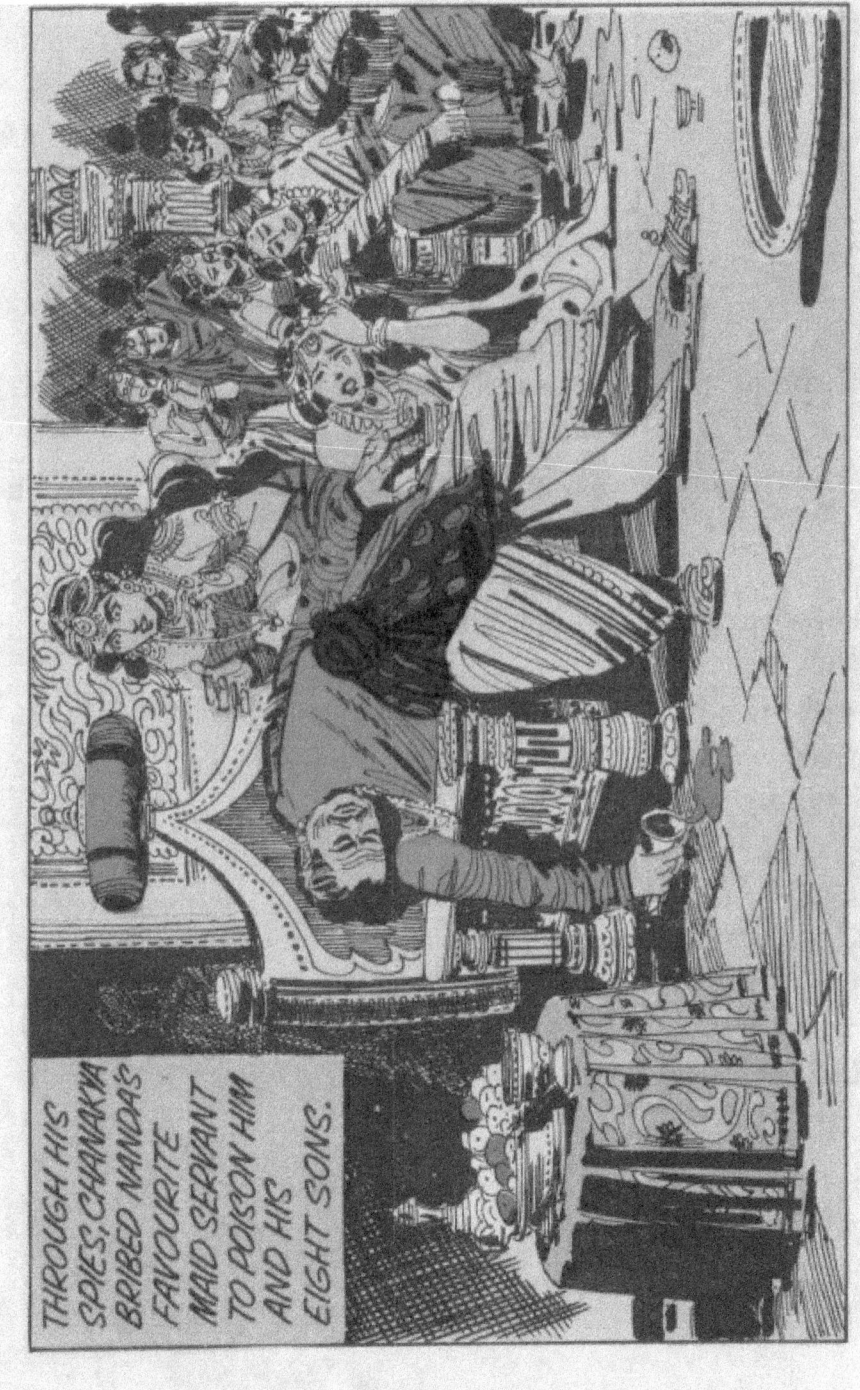

THROUGH HIS SPIES, CHANAKYA BRIBED NANDA'S FAVOURITE MAID SERVANT TO POISON HIM AND HIS EIGHT SONS.

SKILL TO HEAL

Chandragupta's life was at risk after he became the king!

Now Chandragupta was the new king and with Chanakya as his advisor, his strength increased day by day.

But with new victories, Chandragupta made new and deadly enemies also.

Chanakya assessed the danger; he even thought that the new king might even be poisoned to death.

Acharya Chanakya skilled to save from letting killedsaved Chandragupta from poisoning attempt, by his treating doctor, who laced poison, in king's medications.

Source: Pai, Anant. Chanakya: Amar Chitra Katha. Volume 508. India Book House Pvt Ltd. 1971

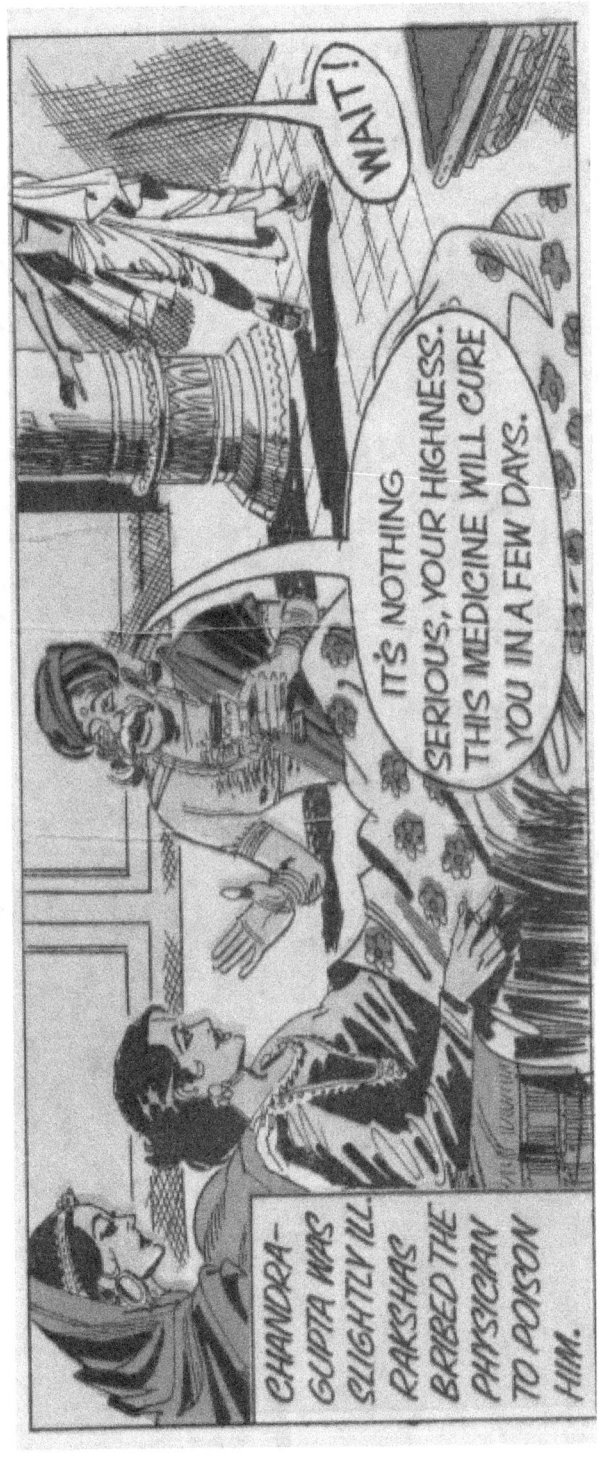

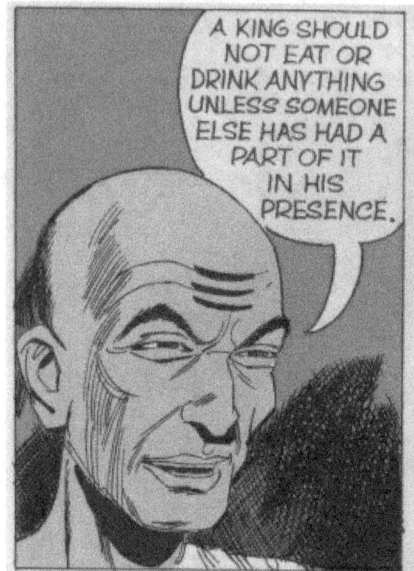

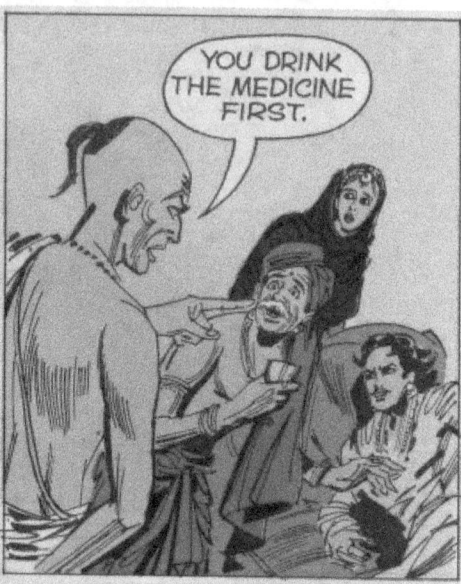

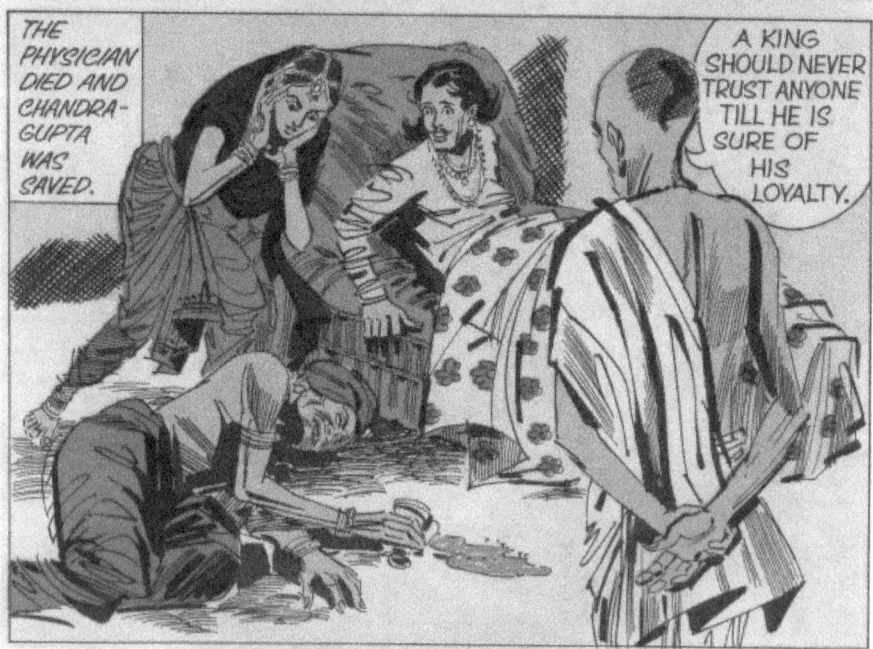

CHANAKYA

: As Indian Mithridates

Did you know that Chanakya was deliberately poisoning in low & slow doses to his king Chandragupta everyday, not to kill him, but to save his life from his enemies!

That's why Chanakya decided to add a pinch of poison to Chandragupta's food to increase his tolerance to the future poisoning attempts by the enemies.

This phenomenon is scientifically now known as drug (toxin) **tolerance:** seen in opium & Arsenic.

But neither Chandragupta nor the queen were aware of this strategy of Chanakya.

Chandragupta, who was not aware of this, once shared the food with his pregnant queen, who was seven days away from delivery.

POISON MAIDEN

Nanda's prime minister Rakshasa escaped Pataliputra, and continued resisting the invaders.

He sent a vishakanya (poison girl) to assassinate Chandragupta.

Chanakya had this girl assassinate Parvata instead, with the blame going to Rakshasa.

Parvata is identified with King Porus by some scholars.

Vishkanya was sent to kill King Chandragupta by Amartya Rakshas, but Acharya Chanakya saved him cleverly, but redirecting the vishkanya to his rival king Parvata.

Motilal Banarsidass (1993). "The Minister Cāṇakya, from the Pariśiṣṭaparvan of Hemacandra". In Phyllis Granoff (ed.). The Clever Adulteress and Other Stories: A Treasury of Jaina Literature. Translated by Rosalind Lefeber. pp. 204–206.

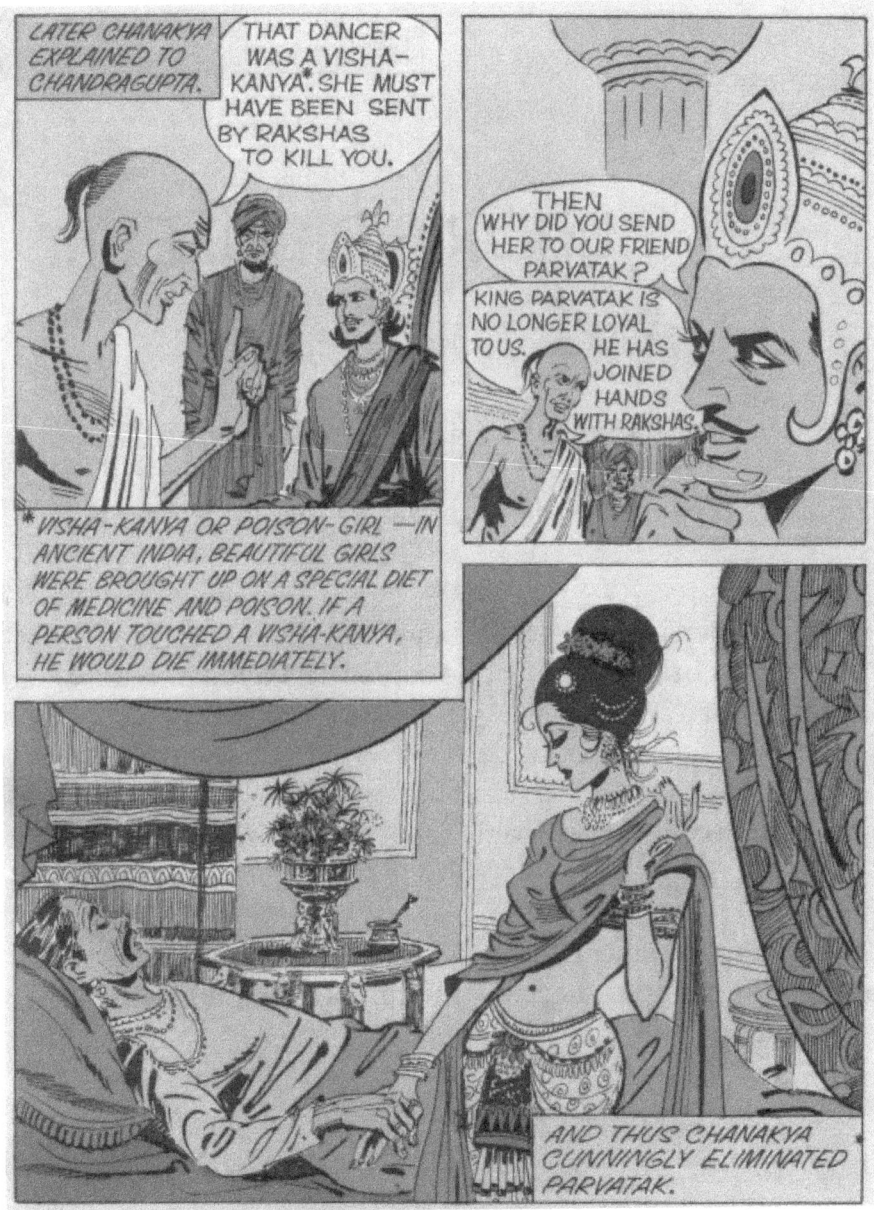

Source: Pai, Anant. Chanakya: Amar Chitra Katha. Volume 508. India Book House Pvt Ltd. 1971

EMPEROR'S RIDDLES

History meets Mystery

This novel features popular episodes from Chanakya's life.

It is a mystery thriller debut novel by Indian author Satyarth Nayak.

The novel consists of a present-day trail of cryptic riddles scattered across India that must be solved one by one to unveil an ancient Indian secret.

This journey plays out in the context of an esoteric legend involving one of the most iconic Emperors of the history of India.

The riddles in the thriller based on Indian history and mythology also become successively complicated and difficult to heighten the mystery.

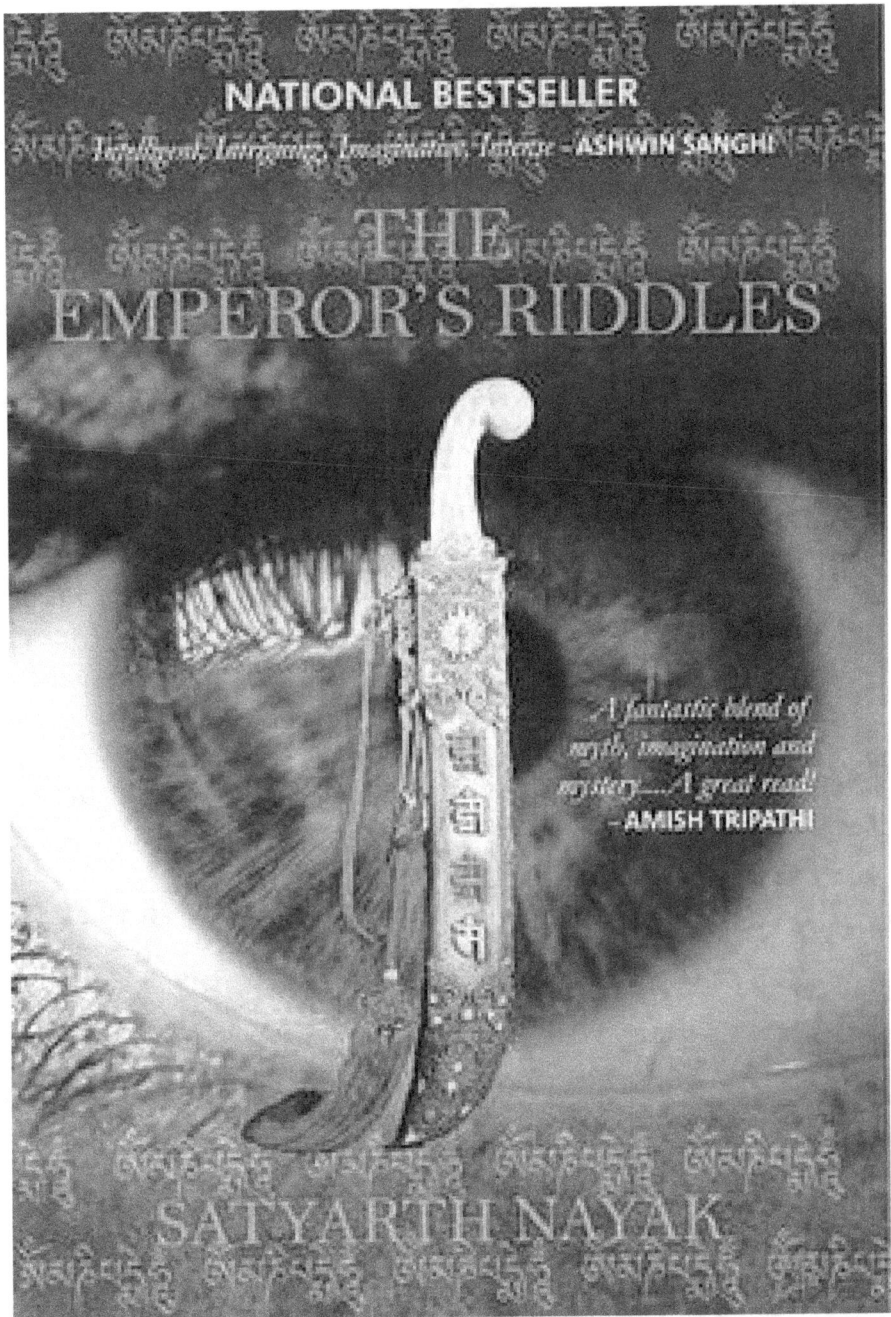

The human quest for answers is the central theme of the book.

The characters are on a personal quest and the final destination may or may not be as per their expectations.

More than the answers, it's the pursuit itself that matters.

Where one riddle ends, another begins.

The novel Emperor's Riddles opens with the bizarre murder of historian at the Ganga ghat in Varanasi.

As his daughter, her close friend, and TV producer investigate the killing, they find a series of cryptic riddles scattered across the country that they must crack one by one to reach a final enigma.

Meanwhile, Chief Officer and journalist are chasing the killer branded as "Scorpion" by the media due to his choice of weapon, a **poisoned syringe**.

At the same time a holy Buddhist Bhikkhu urges his young Samanera Tathagata to make an important journey that promises to alter his life.

Parallel to this is a second storyline which tells the story of the life of a young prince in Ancient India who becomes one of the most celebrated Emperors in history, and who envisions a secret project which could affect the entire world.

The idea for The Emperor's Riddles was born out of a random Internet search by author after reading the Dan Brown thriller Angels & Demons to find out if there was something similarly esoteric and mysterious hidden in the history of India.

"If Brown has codes, my book has riddles."

The surfing yielded an obscure but fascinating conspiracy theory involving one of the greatest Emperors of ancient India.

Author was intrigued by the Emperor's legend and the imperial secret believed to be still alive and functioning and decided to capture this story

KALKI PURANA

A Hindu mythology text, the Kalki Purana, mentions that they can kill a person just by looking at them, and talks about a Visha Kanya named Sulochana, the wife of a Gandharva, Chitragreeva.

The Sri Kalki Purana is a prophetic work in Sanskrit that details the life and times of Kalki, the tenth and final of the Dashavatara of the Hindu deity Lord Vishnu.

The narrative is set near the end of the Kali Yuga or Dark Age, as revealed by the storyteller Suta.

Chaturvedi, BK. Kalki Purana. Diamond Pocket Books (P) Ltd. (2004). p. 74. ISBN 978-81-288-0588-2.

However, in time, "poison damsel" passed into folklore, became an archetype explored by many writers, resulting in a popular literary character that appears in many works, including classical Sanskrit texts such as Sukasaptati.

Śukasaptati, or Seventy tales of the parrot, is a collection of stories originally written in Sanskrit.

The stories are supposed to be narrated to a woman by her pet parrot, at the rate of one story every night, in order to dissuade her from going out to meet her paramour when her husband is away.

Mathur, GL. Erotic Indian tales from the Sanskrit classic Suksaptati, Hind Pocket Books, 1971. Page 26–27.

The Poison Damsel (Sanskrit Viṣakanyā) is a literary figure that appears in Sanskrit literature as a type of assassin used by kings to destroy enemies.

The story goes that young girls were raised on a carefully crafted diet of poison and antidote from a very young age, a practice referred to as mithridatism.

Although many would not survive, those that did were immune to other poisons and their body fluids would be poisonous to others; sexual contact would thus be lethal to other humans.

There also exists a myth that says a Visha Kanya can cause instant death with just a touch.

Since past, these chosen females, who were found to be hyper secretors of toxins fed to them, got trained, for killing their royal victims tactfully. Opium was one of the most common toxins given for killing precious royal princes mostly for infanticide.

In Indian Mythology, Demon Pootana was, one of the Poison Damsel, who tried to kill infantile Lord Krishna.

IS THERE ANY SCIENTIFIC HYPOTHESIS FOR TOXIC ASSASSINS IN REALITY?

Is it possible, to feed a chosen animal first, on the toxin in low doses, and gradually increase it chronically, till the tolerance develops, and that animal can ingest large doses later, without any toxic effects.

But when, this first animal is sent to co-habit with another animal, to stay in close physical contact for days, and the first animal still keeps on consuming the toxin secretly, but the second animal in first's close association, develops its acute toxicity, due to secondary exposure to the culprit toxin in fatal dose actually & dies suddenly.

And the first animal, walks out, safely.

As the chosen ones were ultra-rapid metabolizer of opium.

These Poisoners might have multiple duplications of specific cytochrome P450 metabolizing opioids in their body.

Discovering these toxicological mysteries, hidden in our ancient mythology, with logical hypothesis on scientific basis, decoding myths, is the clue to solve these riddles.

45

Toxic Riddle in Rhymes;
Pin Doll with pointed nail;

Ox on snuffs & sail;

Notorious serial killer, tempt;

In repeated heinous contempt;

Sent selected Poisoner for homicidal attempt;

An incarnate enemy of fragile status, in week;

Poisoning by specifics was the commonest strategy, to peek;

Killing this generation, before they might speak;

Poisoners were loaded, trained & hired

for killing precious enemies, seek;

Several of the physicians suspected these poisoners as unique;

And Centuries later, were scientifically able

to explain, language similar to greek;

That the chosen ones would been ultra-rapid metabolizer, chic;

As Poisoner might have multiple duplications

of specifics's cytochrome P450 peak;

Instead of converting the normal

5% to 10% of soothers to anodynes, leak;

Poisoner would be converting nearly

all of the toxic nostrums, collected in streak;

Multiple serial cases of lethal intoxication had been

reported since antiquity, to sneak;

Guess the toxin, toxic methodology & solve

the toxic riddle into plique;

45 RIDDLE ANALYSIS

In past, chosen females, who were found to be secretors of opium toxicity, got trained, for killing tactfully. Opium was the most common toxin given for infanticide.

The Visha Kanya (Sanskrit विष कन्या; English: Poison girl) were young women reportedly used as assassins, often against powerful enemies, during the times of the Ancient India.

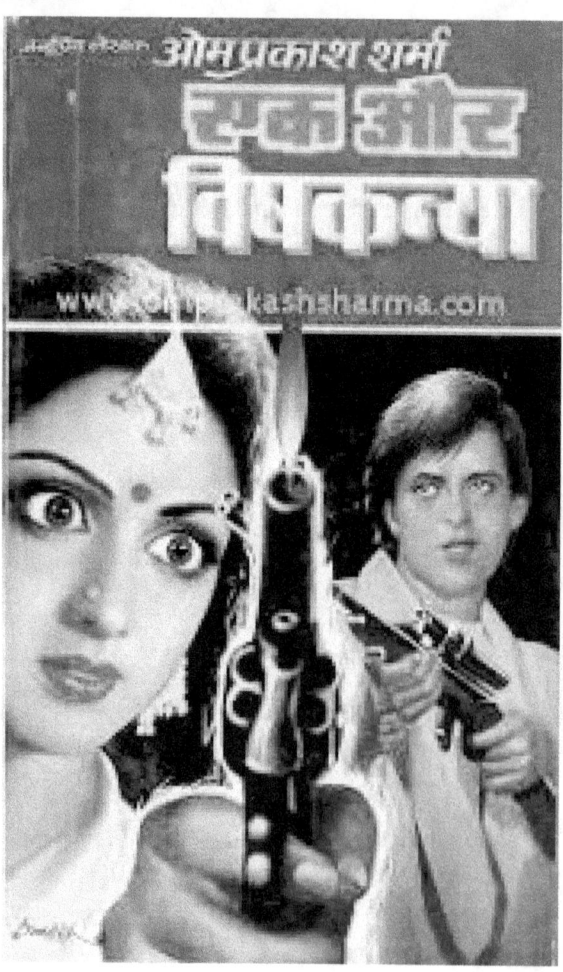

Visha Kanya has been a popular theme in Indian literature and folklore, and apart from appearing in classical Sanskrit texts, it has appeared repeatedly in various works like Vishkanya by Shivani and Ek Aur Vish Kanya? by Om Prakash Sharma, who use Visha Kanya as an archetype in their stories—a beautiful girl who kills when she comes too close.

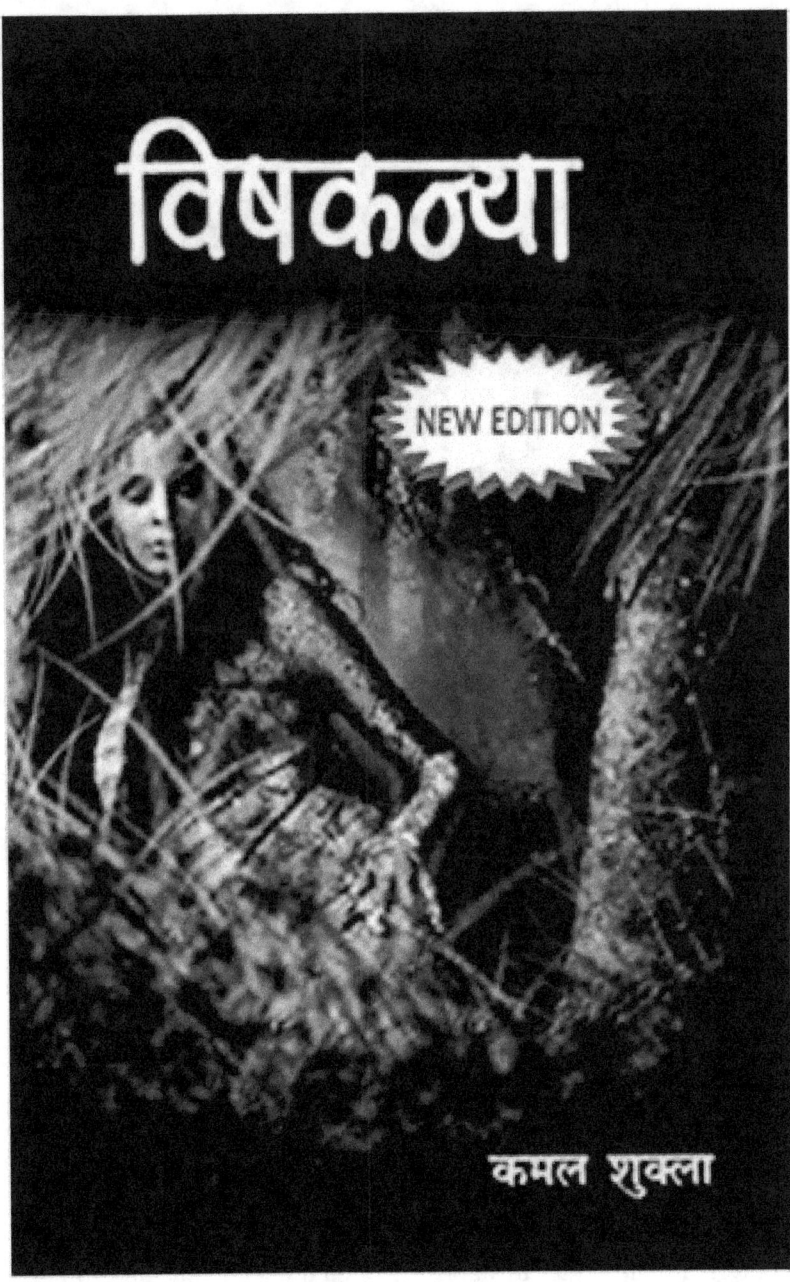

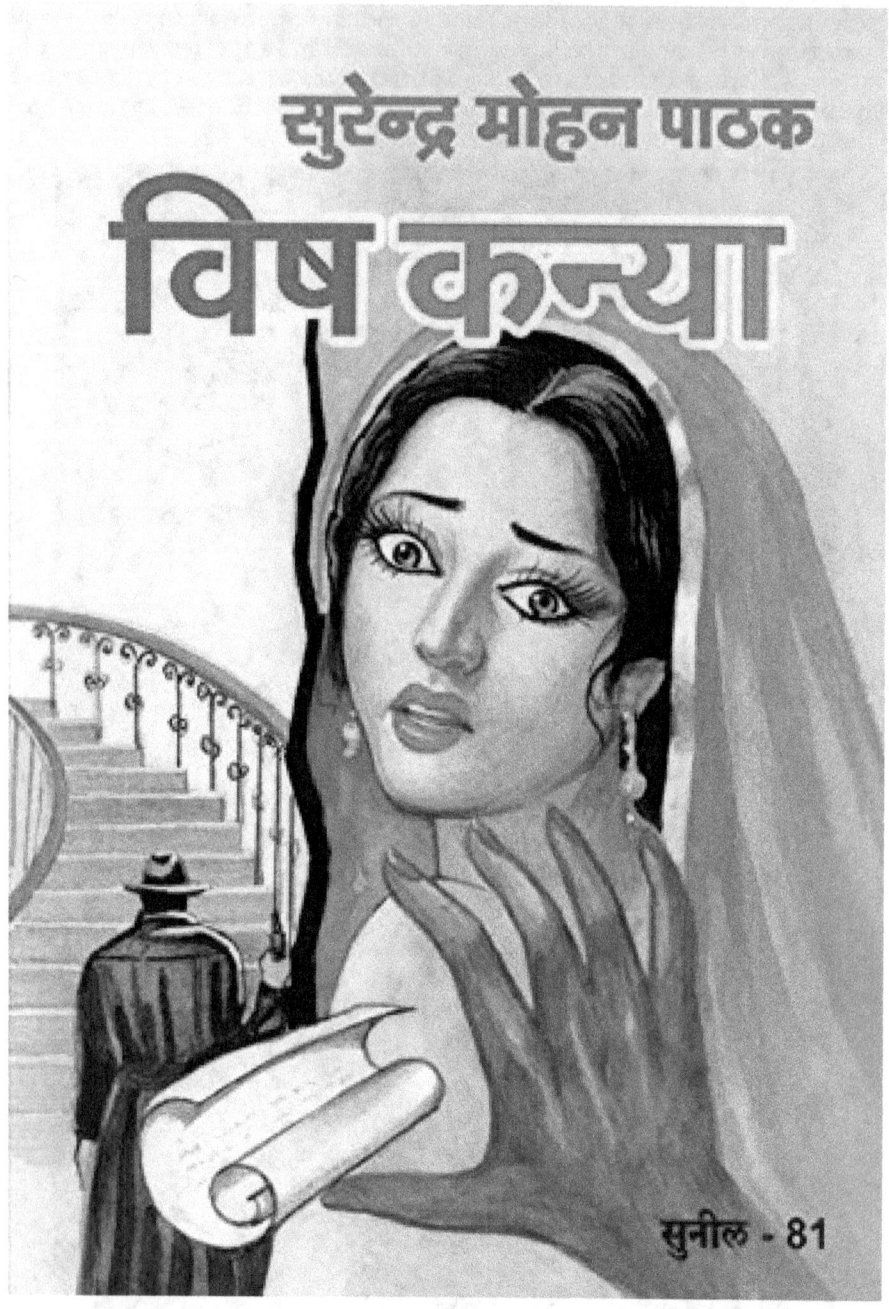

More recently, the archetype has taken a new hue in the HIV/AIDS era, for example in Vishkanya, a 2007 novel, based on the AIDS epidemic in society.

In 2009, Vibha Rahi, a lower caste woman has written an autobiography 'Vishkanya: Untold Secrets' in Marathi, in which she portrays how upper caste women make intimate relationships with lower caste people of high profile and destroy their families and social relationships.

Rahi, Vibha (2009). Vishkanya: Untold Secrets. Pune: Karuvaki Prakashan.

Obviously, the issue with these stories is they are fiction and no authentic sources confirm any of them. They need check from other chronicled sources.

PIN DOLL WITH POINTED NAIL, OX ON SNUFFS & SAIL;

Victim (the infant), once intoxicated, behaves like doll, don't breath, don't move, feel cold to touch in suspended animation.

Doll's eye movement

Doll's don't wake up, Pin the doll with pointed nail.

Pin point pupil

Nail- Ox-on side snuffs & sail

(naloxone) inject on biceps or inhale puff in one side.

DOLL'S EYE MOVEMENT

The oculocephalic reflex (doll's eyes reflex) is an application of the vestibular-ocular reflex (VOR) used for neurologic examination of cranial nerves 3, 6, and 8, the reflex arc including brainstem nuclei, and overall gross brainstem function.

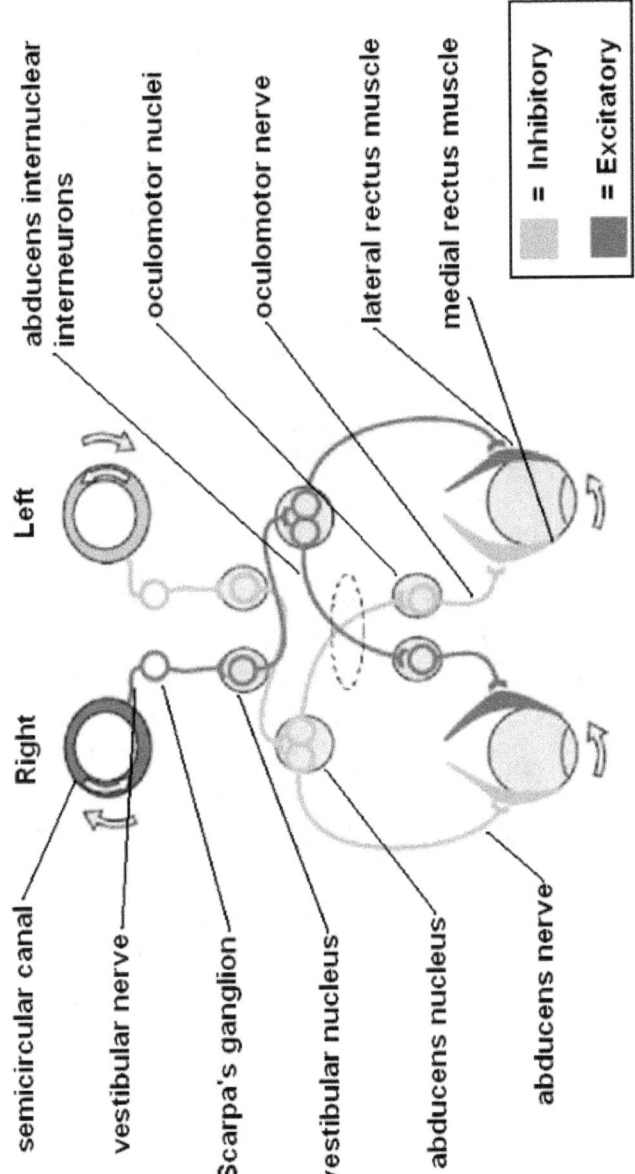

Figure 1. Vestibulo-ocular reflex. Courtesy: https://commons.wikimedia.org/wiki/File:Vestibulo-ocular_reflex.PNG

The reflex is suppressed in a conscious adult with normal neurologic function but is active in a comatose patient with gross brainstem function, absent if there is damage to the reflex arc.

Sharshar T, et al. Paris-Ouest Study Group on Neurological Effect of Sedation (POSGNES). Brainstem responses can predict death and delirium in sedated patients in intensive care unit. Crit. Care Med. 2011 Aug;39(8):1960-7.

It is often used to examine patients in the neurologic critical care setting but also may have utility to assess neonates, anesthetized patients, or dizzy patients.

Neonates - Most neonates exhibit an unsuppressed doll's eyes reflex before 11.5 weeks; this can serve as a neonatal milestone in neurologic development.

Snir M, et al. Suppression of the oculocephalic reflex (doll's eyes phenomenon) in normal full-term babies. Curr. Eye Res. 2010 May;35(5):370-4.

The reflex derives its name from the characteristic doll's eyes appearance that a patient has if the reflex is positive.

The oculocephalic reflex is performed by holding a patient's eyelids open and moving their head from side to side.

The examination should only be performed on patients with a stable cervical spine without c-spine precautions.

With the patient's eyelids open, the examiner briskly rotates the patient's head from side to side while the examiner observes the patient's eyes.

The examiner observes a positive oculocephalic reflex when the patient moves their eyes opposite of the rotation of their head, such that their eyes stay looking forward (like a doll's eyes).

The examiner observes a negative oculocephalic reflex when the patient's eyes stay midline and do not move while the examiner rotates the head.

NOTORIOUS SERIAL KILLER, TEMPT;

According to the Indian Arthashastra, Vish kanya was allegedly used by Nanda Dynasty founder Mahapadma Nanda to kill the last ruler of Shishunaga Dynasty Kalashoka both of which belonged to mighty Magadha Kingdom

Visha Kanya was allegedly sent by Nanda's minister Amatyarakshasa to kill Chandragupta Maurya and Chanakya diverted them to kill Parvatak.

The name 'Visha Kanya' comes from the Sanskrit for 'poison girl' or 'poison damsel' – a literal description of the role of the Visha Kanya who were female assassins who killed with poison.

The group began between 340 and 293 BC when they were set up by the first Indian Maurya Emperor, Chandragupta.

Their utilization by the state was recorded in the Arthashastra, a manual of statecraft written by Chanakya, the prime minister of the emperor.

The Arthashastra recommended that the Emperor needed to maintain a network of agents to monitor and manipulate his enemies. Assassination was a form of covert war, and to that end, the King needed to retain operatives who could deal with specific targets. These agents were not just men. They also included women.

"To undermine a ruling oligarchy, make chiefs of the [enemy's] ruling council infatuated with women possessed of great beauty and youth, " advised Chanakya, " When passion is roused in them, they should start quarrels by creating belief (about their love) in one and by going to another." (Arthashastra 11.1).

This is where the Vishakanya came in.

However, although noted for their beauty, they were not just deployed to cause fights between love rivals; they killed their potential lovers.

The training of a Vishakanya began as a child. After recruitment, each girl was fed a modulated diet of poison.

This practice, known as Mithridatism was designed to render the future assassin immune to the poison they would use on their targets.

This meant the Vishakanya could administer poison directly, perhaps even tasting it themselves to divert suspicion before – and after – the kill.

Many girls did not survive the training, as they could not withstand preparatory dosage.

Those that did were sent out in their King's service in the guise of courtesans.

So legendary was the skill of the Vishakanya, it was believed their bodily fluids were naturally poisonous so that even a kiss from them was death.

In all probability, the girl's administered the poison in other ways, using alcohol or food as a carrier. This way, they could share the tainted feasts with their targets, safe because of their immunity.

Norman Mosley Penzer; Somadeva Bhatta (November 1980). Poison-damsels: Folklore of the World. Ayer Publishing. p. 17. ISBN 978-0-405-13336-7.

VISHKANYA & SANKHYA

traditional name of toxic arsenic salt- संख्या

Chronic low dose of arsenic makes person tolerant to high doses.

So Arsenophagists can survive toxic dose of arsenic.

Vish-kanya were Arsenophagists, who were sent to assassinate the enemy king by applying arsenic on skin, hair & nails.

When the targeted enemy enjoyed with vishkanya & share arsenic toxicated drink with vishkanya, the enemy dies but vishkanya survived for future use.

How to easy Recall Arsenic (संख्या- count)– (बाल- BAL)- uses, misuse, signs & symptoms, diagnosis, detection & treatment

संख्या- used traditionally as disinfectant to save ऊन के बाल from parasites - in Sheep farming for getting wools.

बाल- "unlimited" hair- in counting – संख्या- sankya- traditional name of toxic arsenic salt as it kills uncountable in small dose.

बाल- "unlimited" hair- Mass poisoning- Unlimited संख्या victims – drinking well poisoned killing unlimited.

बाल- "unlimited" hair – Unlimited संख्या Loose motions- Rice water Stool- can see rice-size white hair(बाल) "unlimited" संख्या -small mucosal pieces floating in stool of enteritis victim poisoned by संख्या.

बाल- killer- Abortifacient- killing unborn child by संख्या poison.

Chronic repeated dose- deposit in hair (बाल)- can be detected in alive & dead victim's hair.

Chronic repeated dose- deposit in Nails- horizontal white thin hair- like- बाल- Aldrich Mees' lines.

Chronic repeated dose- Skin – raindrops pigmentation- rain – unlimited count (संख्या) drops.

Lab- White Blood counts- संख्या- increased in संख्या poisoning- Leukocytosis, relative eosinophilia.

Lab- Red Blood counts- संख्या- decreases rapidly in संख्या poisoning- Normocytic Anemia due to hemolysis, hematuria, GI bleed.

Lab- Platelet counts- संख्या- decreases rapidly in संख्या poisoning – thrombo-cytopenia.

Postmortem- Stomach shows red velvet carpet appearance in संख्या poisoning- बाल- unlimited count- संख्या red short बाल 'hair- like' carpet on stomach- due to mucosal damage & congestion by irritant संख्या

Antidote- बाल- BAL(British Anti Lewsite)- Dimercaprol. Chelation therapy- बाल चिपकना- Antidote sticks to Arsenic & neutralizes its toxicity.

Arsenic Can be detected even after cremation (बाल-दो)- burning poisoned to destroy evidence.

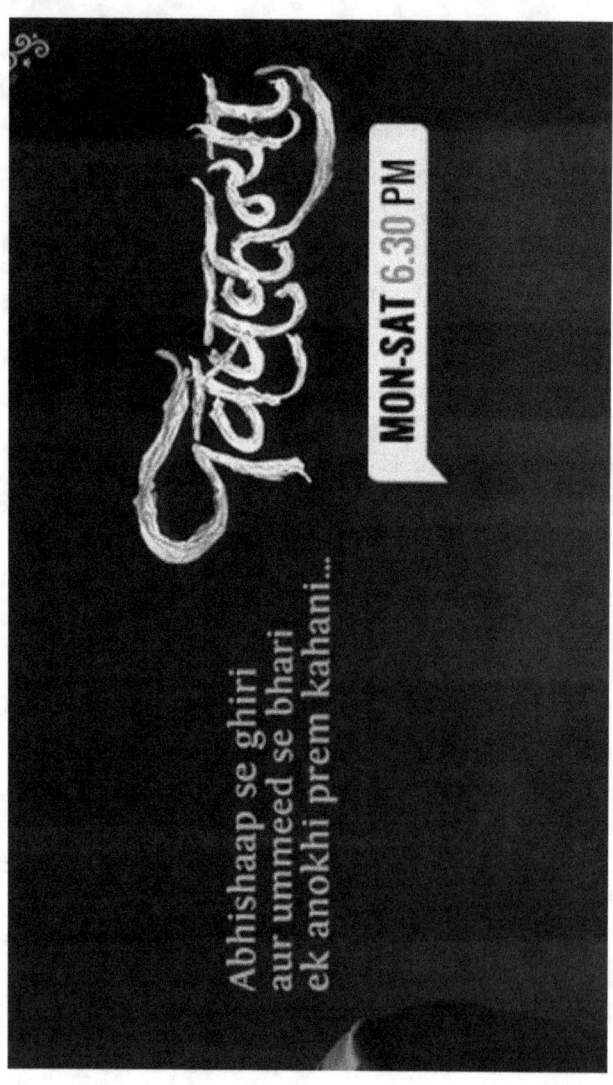

IN REPEATED
HEINOUS CONTEMPT;

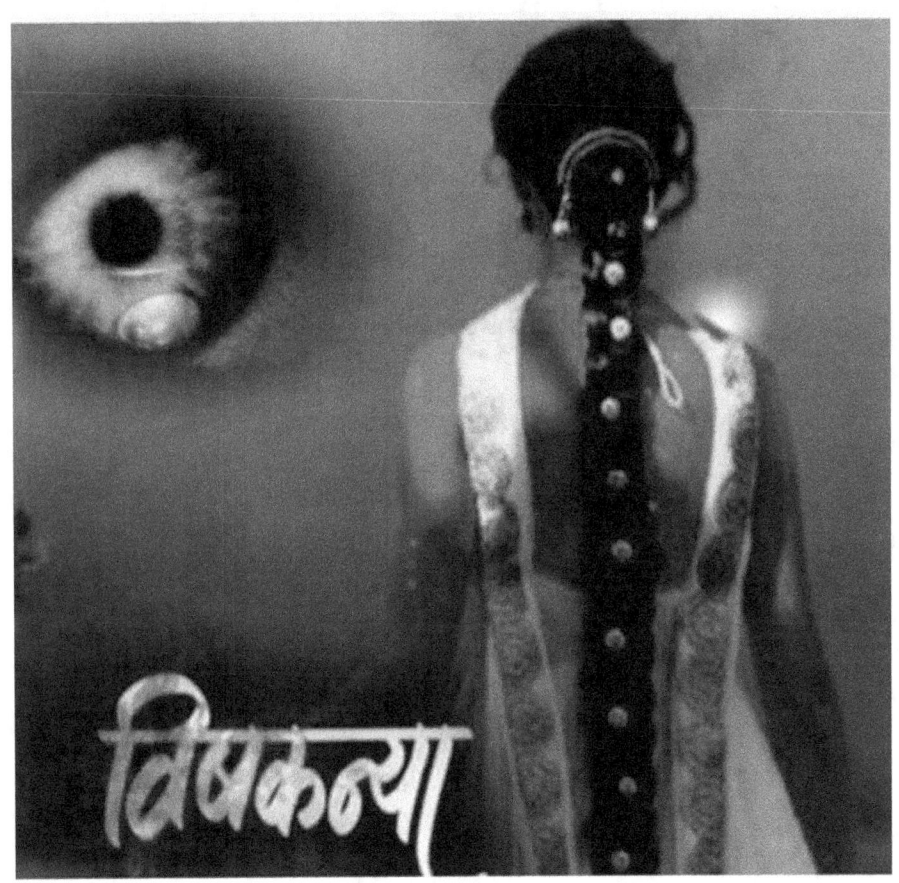

SENT SELECTED POISONER FOR HOMICIDAL ATTEMPT;

Pootna was selected by demon King Kans, to kill Lord Krishna

AN INCARNATE ENEMY OF FRAGILE STATUS, IN WEEK;

Talking about Lord Krishna, the incarnation of Lord Vishnu, as per Bhagwat Purnana.

POISONING BY SPECIFICS WAS THE COMMONEST STRATEGY, TO PEEK;

Opium posioning is the most common type of toxin used for infanticide all over the world

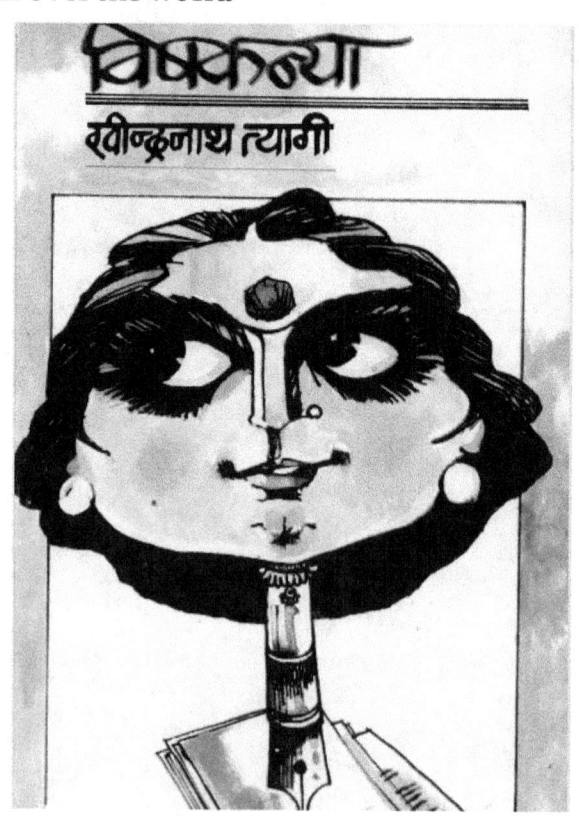

KILLING THIS GENERATION, BEFORE THEY MIGHT SPEAK;

As the infants are imbecile & can't speak & blame, who poisoned them, so poisoning is more common

POISONERS WERE LOADED, TRAINED & HIRED FOR KILLING PRECIOUS ENEMIES, SEEK;

Vishkanyas are a race of exotic humanoids with poisonous blood.

Vishkanya, actually signifying "lady with poison", originates from sources in which old Indian

Kings prepared young ladies to kill their enemies , When these ladies achieved pubescence, they

would become completely lethal and prepared to be used as savage human weapons.

Indeed, even a touch of them can kill someone.

Be that as it may, nobody can state for certain where truth closures and myth starts about the accuracy of these venomous professional killers.

Aristotle, the great thinker cautioned Alexander the Great about the perils of such "venomous virgins" before the Alexander, the great Greek King propelled his Indian crusade.

Another Indian legend even recommends that Alexander the Great died because of a Vishkanya that was sent to him as a trophy by the crushed King Porus.

Possessed of an alien beauty, these graceful humanoids see the world through serpentine eyes of burnished gold. Their supple skin is covered with tiny scales, often of a light green, which are sometimes arrayed in patterns not unlike those of a serpent. They cannot be generalized as good or evil, but since they truly speak with forked tongues, they are content to accept the gold they're offered and leave questions of morality to others.

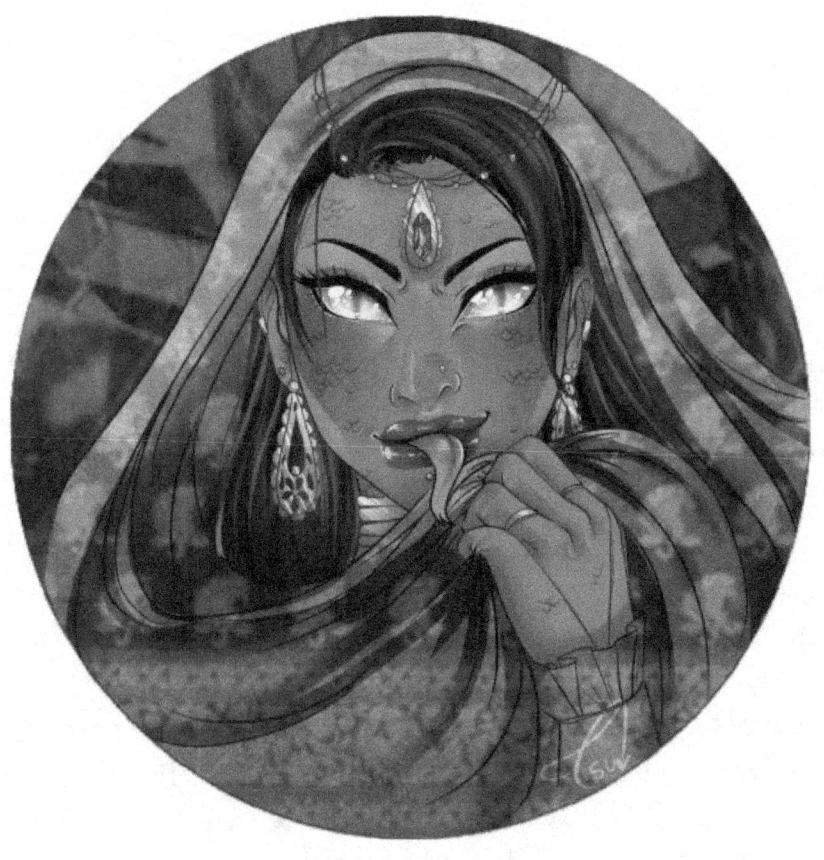

BASIC INSTINCT

Honey Trap

The human need for food and sex are basic, part of the foundation of our nature, which makes it sensible that they are so closely knit together.

That need is misued to assasinate the royal princes, who were humans too, thus falling prey to the honey trap, of poison maidens.

As desire for sexual attraction develops only after age of puberty, due to hormonal surge, so killers used to honey trap laced with poison in the basic food of targeted infants, that is the breast milk.

As per Bhagwat Purana in Indian Mythology, infamous Poison Maiden: **Pootana** was hired, one of the Poison Damsels trained by Mathura King, who tried to kill infantile Lord Krishna, by suckling breast filled with opium rich milk.

But this bonding & likeness for mother's breast remains whole life in the psychology of most humans, till they die.

In all cultures, men manipulated manually (98%) and orally (93%) the breast of their partners & do suck it like a child.

Citation: Dixson BJ, Duncan M, Dixson AF. The Role of Breast Size and Areolar Pigmentation in Perceptions of Women's Sexual Attractiveness, Reproductive Health, Sexual Maturity, Maternal Nurturing Abilities, and Age. Arch Sex Behav. 2015 Aug;44(6):1685-95.

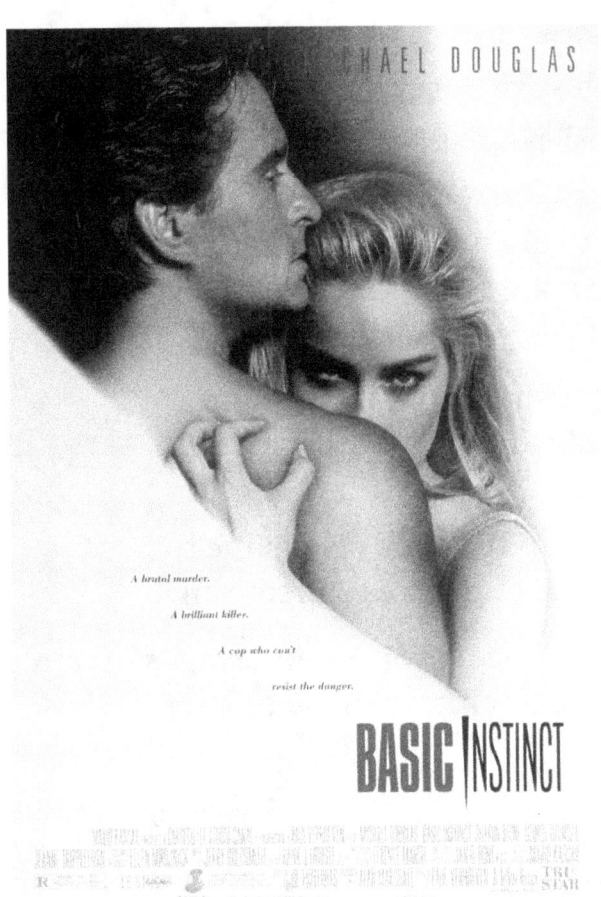

This fondness for human breast might have been the basic mechanism of assassinating by Poison Maidens.

This suckling is nature's way of feeding the infant, but in adults, it transferred the toxic contents of the breast of poison maidens, in form of the milk into the targeted enemy's body via oral route, intoxicating him, thus making him sedated, obtundated, comatose and vulnerable to die.

People who are obtunded have a more depressed level of consciousness and cannot be fully aroused.

Those who are not able to be aroused from a sleep-like state are said to be stuporous.

Coma is the inability to make any purposeful response.

Thus dying in his deep sleep, due to hypoxia, due to failure to breath in.

This is the typical progression stages of narcosis to coma, seen with opium & opiates.

Coma literally means, just before ending the sentence.

Thus medically coma is the last stage,

just before ending the life.

I t's a hypothesis, based on the journal referenced, please excuse us, for being so explicit in explaining, but most of assassins kept their methods hidden, and thus analysis is retrograde extrapolation, with the available information from that time.

Since opium was rampantly available, and genetic mechanism for its rapid metabolisers, might have played important role, in developing toxic assassins, from innocent & harmless looking, young females, attractive for seduction.

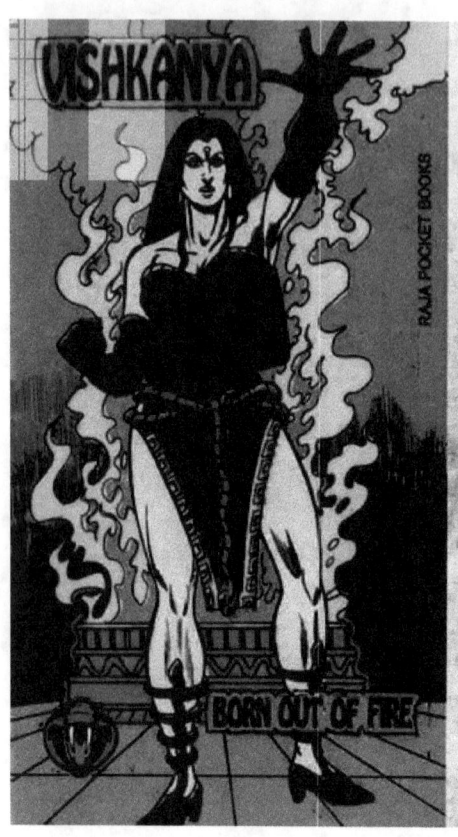

डियर कलेक्टर,

राजतांत्रिक विषंधर ने यक्षराक्षस गरलगंट को देव कालजयी के विष से बुझे फ्लों की आहुति देकर प्रगट होने के लिए विवश कर दिया था, जिसकी इच्छा थी नागराज को खत्म करने की शक्ति पैदा करना । जिसके परिणामस्वरूप प्रगट हुई एक ऐसी शक्ति के रूप में मैं जिसके पास नागराज की हरेक शक्ति का जवाब मौजूद था । मुझमें नागराज की समस्त शक्तियों को सोखकर उसका वार उसी पर करने की क्षमता है और मेरे जीवन का उद्देश्य ही नागराज की मौत है । अब मुझे सिर्फ यही देखना है । नागराज मुझसे कब तक बचा रह सकता है?

NAG-39-A-2.9.97

आपकी विषकन्या

Basic Instinct is a 1992 neo-noir erotic thriller film, he film follows San Francisco police detective (Michael Douglas), who is investigating the brutal murder of a wealthy rock star. During the investigation, he becomes involved in a torrid and intense relationship with the prime suspect (Sharon Stone), an enigmatic writer.

SEVERAL OF THE PHYSICIANS SUSPECTED THESE POISONERS AS UNIQUE;

Vishkanya often approach their objectives by alluring them and giving them harmed poison.

They would normally drink poison from the glass to pick up the trust of their casualty and when the clueless casualty would drink from a similar container, he would ingest toxic substance into his body.

Scholars additionally find out about the "Toxic substance Damsel" (Sanskrit Viṣakanyā), that shows up in Sanskrit writing as a kind of professional killer utilized by rulers to murder their foes.

As per the source, young ladies were raised and were made to eat toxic substance from an early age, it was a system known as Mithridatism.

As indicated by the stories, a lot of these young ladies died during the process of making them a Vishkanya, but those who survived , ended up as a human weapon as their organic liquids in body turned out to be to a great toxic to others.

Any contact, particularly sexual contact, was deadly to the men who had the misfortune to lay down with these Vishkanyas.

In any case, in time, "Harm Maid" go into old stories, turned into a paradigm investigated by numerous scholars, bringing about a mainstream abstract character that shows up in numerous works, including traditional Sanskrit, for example, Sukasaptati.

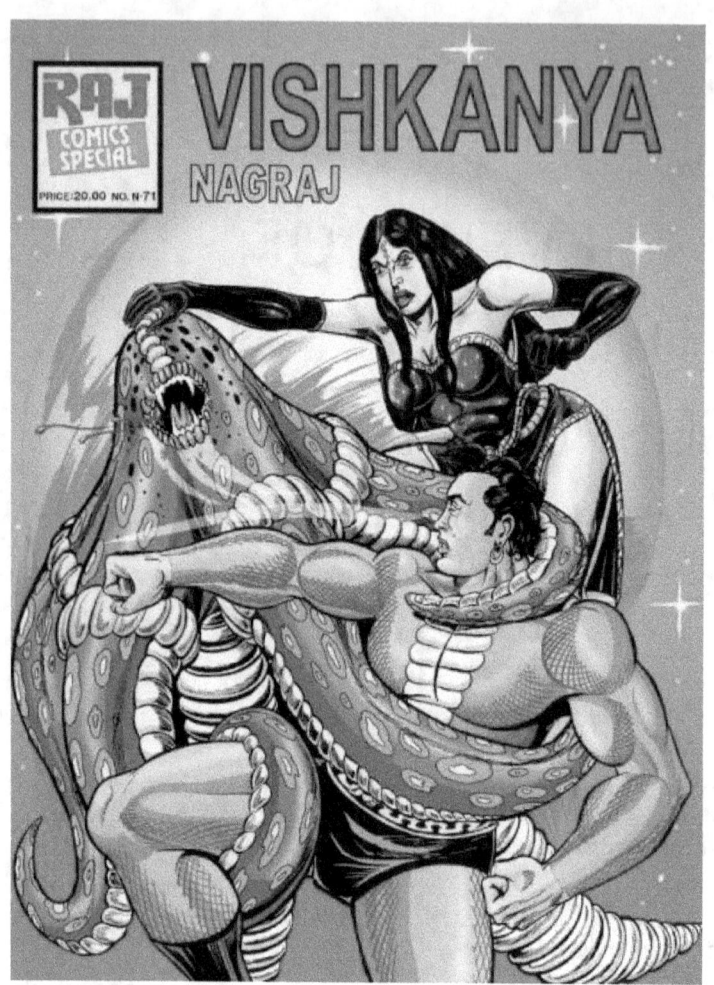

VISH KANYA DOSHA

Astrology talks of a Vish Kanya Dosha (fault) which did not give the couple a happy wedded life. It was presumed as myth that the husband dies prematurely, if the wife has this finding in her Birth chart.

विषकन्या योग = वैधव्य/विधवा

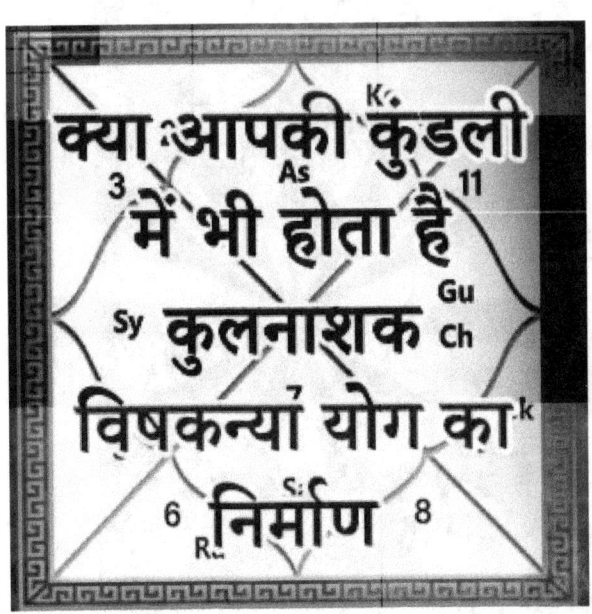

These girls were promised an early widowhood if

they were married. Again, could be a superstition.

These girls were recruited by Kings and Ministers to kill the enemies.

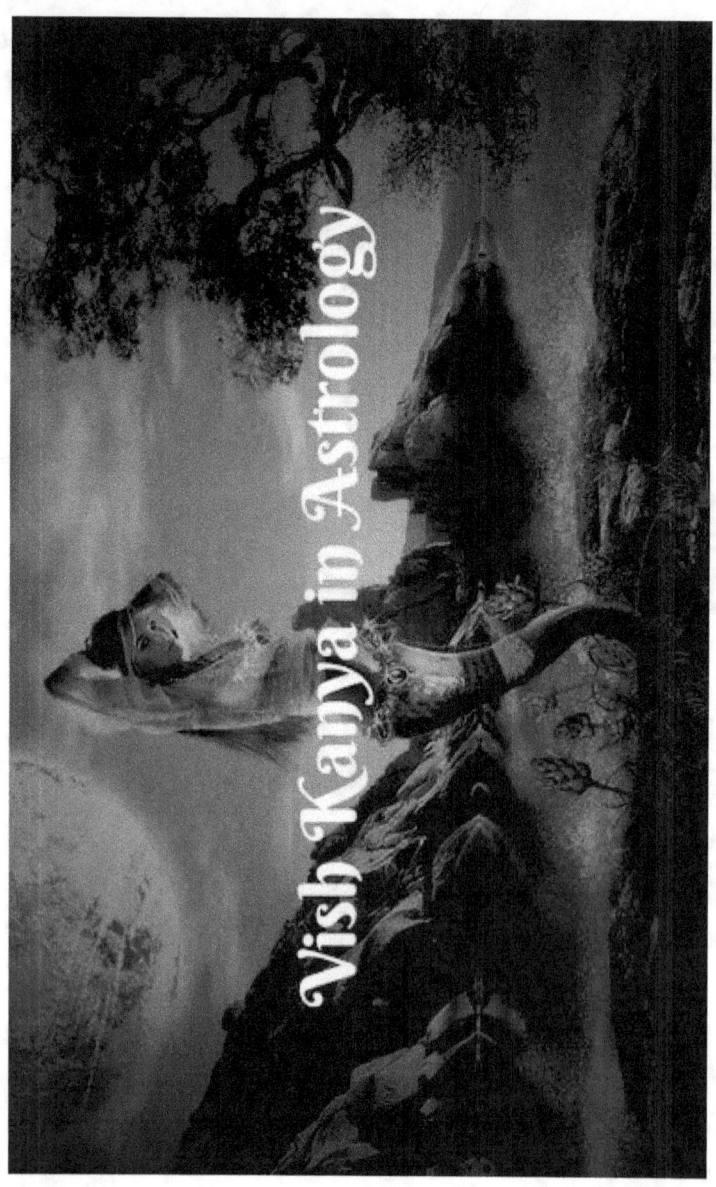

Vish Kanya in Astrology

AND CENTURIES LATER, WERE SCIENTIFICALLY ABLE TO EXPLAIN, LANGUAGE SIMILAR TO GREEK;

Sanskrit & German language are similar to Greek. A Greek study by Dr. Eugenia Yiannakopoulou Department of Medical Laboratories, Faculty of Health and Caring Professions, Technological Educational Institute of Athens, Athens, Greece, hypothesized about Poison damsels.

Citation: Eugenia Y. Pharmacogenomics and Opioid Analgesics: Clinical Implications. International Journal of Genomics Volume 2015, Article ID 368979, 8 pages.

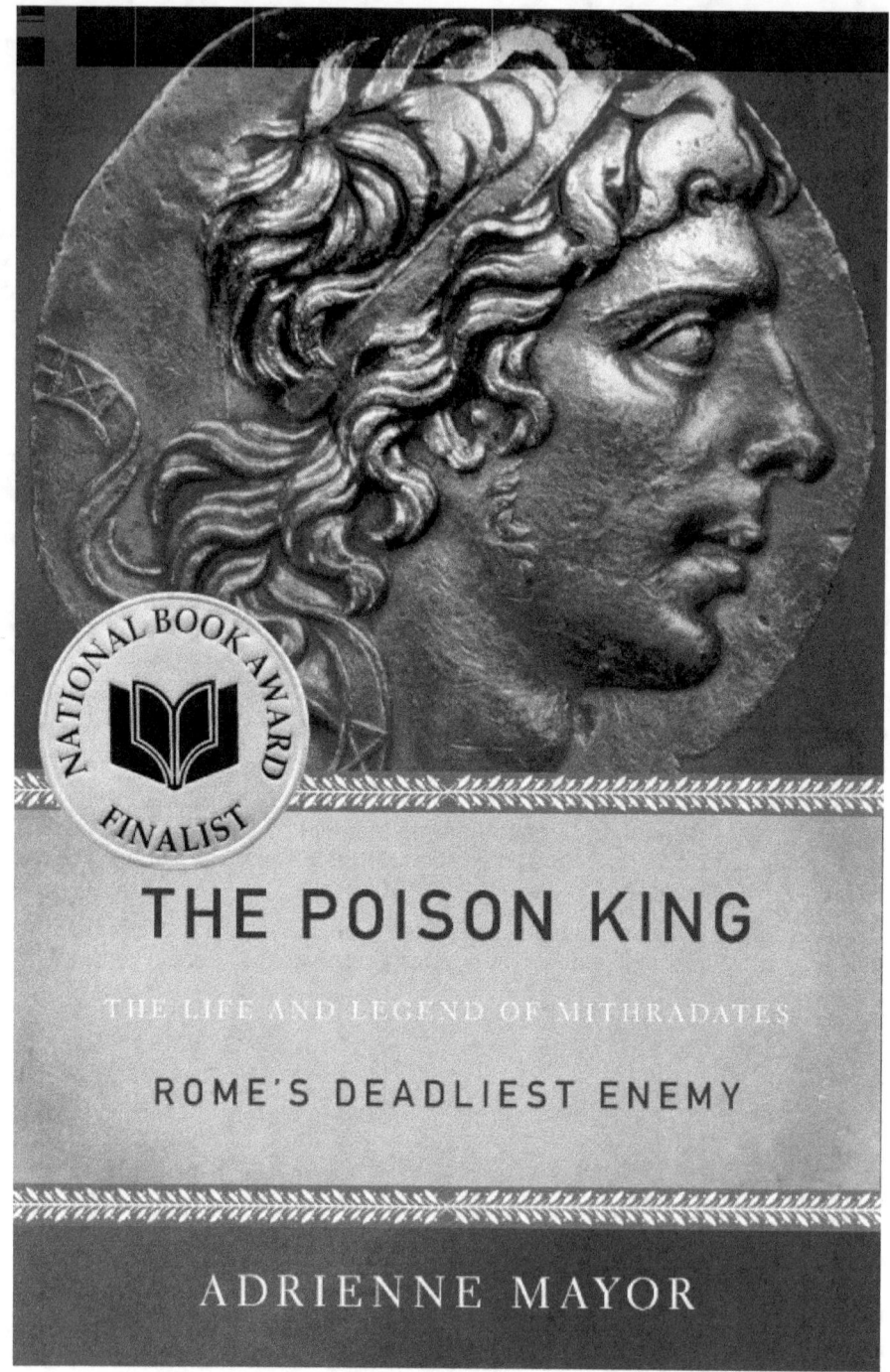

NATIONAL BOOK AWARD FINALIST

THE POISON KING

THE LIFE AND LEGEND OF MITHRADATES

ROME'S DEADLIEST ENEMY

ADRIENNE MAYOR

MITHRIDATISM:

immunity to Poisoning

It depends on the poison, but sometime the process of building up an immunity to poison is referred to as mithridatism, after legends about Greek King Mithridates the sixth.

After his father was poisoned, Mithridates VI decided to subject himself to a daily routine of all-known-poisons to become immune to poison.

Mithridates, king of Pontus (in modern Turkey), lived from 132 to 63 BC and had the reputation of knowing more about poisons and their proper antidotes than any other person of his time.

He was very concerned with the possibility of being assassinated by poison, so he experimented with poisons and antidotes on himself as well as captured prisoners.

He developed a so-called universal antidote, which was called "Mithridatum" in his honor.

This antidote remained so popular in the minds of the people that it was still available in Italian pharmacies up through the 17th century.

Once again, considering the ingredients of this mixture with today's toxicological knowledge, it is obvious that little protection could be obtained from Mithridates' antidote.

Trestrail, JH. Criminal Poisoning- Investigational Guide for Law Enforcement, Toxicologists, Forensic Scientists, and Attorneys. 2nd Ed. Humana Press. 2007.

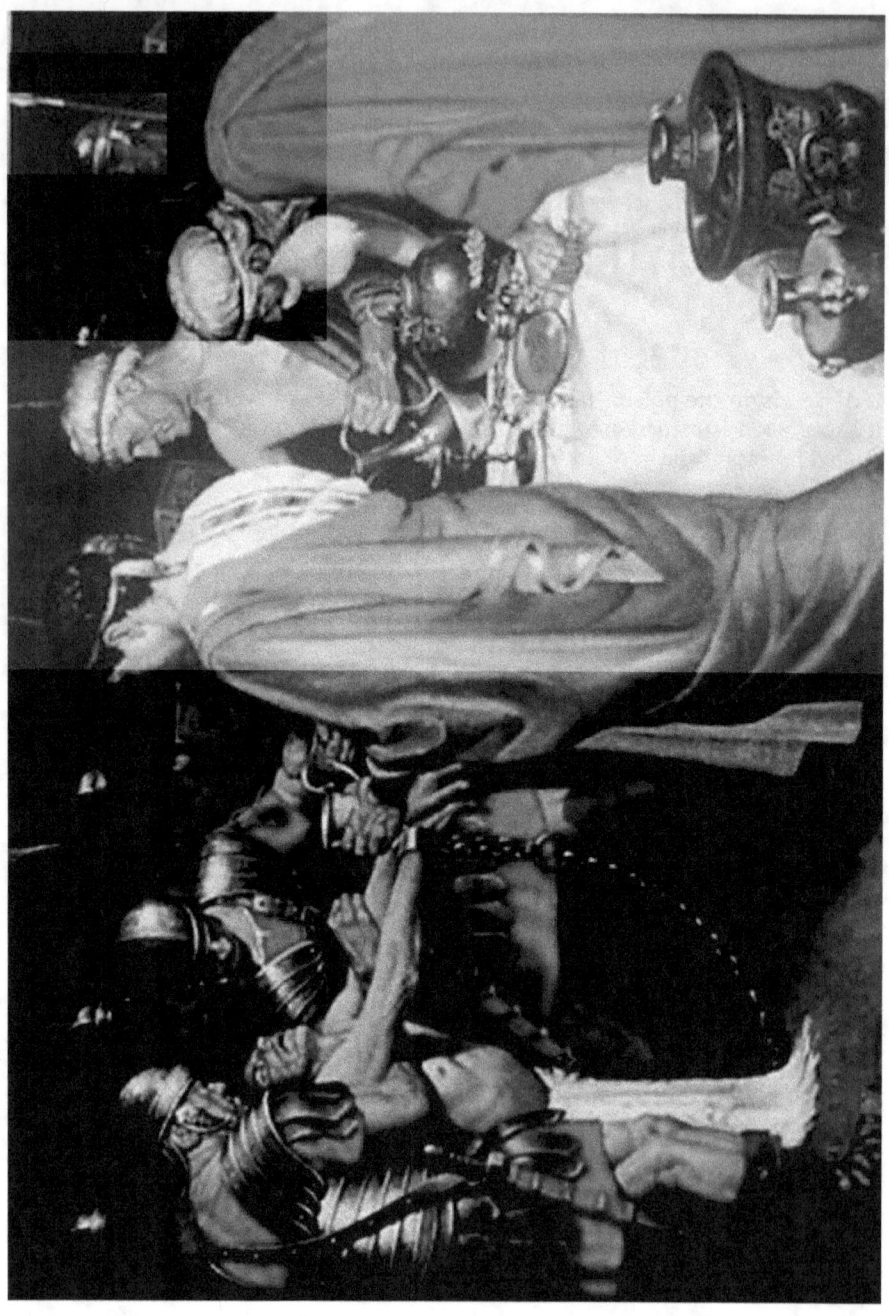

THAT THE CHOSEN ONES WOULD BEEN ULTRA-RAPID METABOLIZER, CHIC;

Chic is a slang word used for complimenting beautiful attractive girl.

AS POISONER MIGHT
HAVE MULTIPLE
DUPLICATIONS
OF SPECIFICS'S
CYTOCHROME
P450 PEAK;

INSTEAD OF CONVERTING THE NORMAL 5% TO 10% OF SOOTHERS TO ANODYNES, LEAK;

Opium was used in past for infants as Soothers, Nostrums & Anodynes

Anodyne properties of certain plants like opium, soothing & sedating to the mind

POISONER WOULD
BE CONVERTING
NEARLY ALL OF THE
TOXIC NOSTRUMS,
COLLECTED IN
STREAK;

MULTIPLE SERIAL CASES OF LETHAL INTOXICATION HAD BEEN REPORTED SINCE ANTIQUITY, TO SNEAK;

Ancient Indian Astrology for match making, describes of a Vish Kanya Dosha (fault) which did not give the couple a happy wedded life.

These girls were promised an early widowhood if they were married, and are called Black Widow.

These people were recruited by Kings and Ministers to kill the enemies.

As mentioned in a Marathi book, "Samrat Akbar" and Persian source by Abdul quadir Badyuni (a account of historian on Akbar) it is stated that sending Vishkanya was a joint conspiracy of Mahachuchak Begum , Mirza Hakim's mother and Abdul Mali', Akbar's brother in law . Abdul Mali sent Vishkanya from Kabul to kill Akbar.

GUESS THE
TOXIN, TOXIC
METHODOLOGY &
SOLVE THE TOXIC
RIDDLE INTO PLIQUE;

MYTHOLOGICAL OPIUM USE TO INFANTICIDE

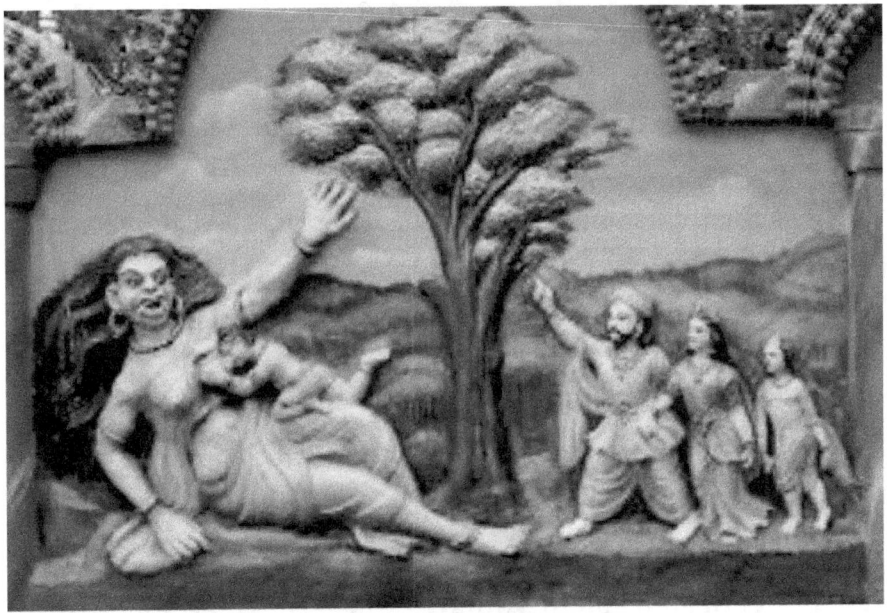

Figure 2. Poison Damsels: Opium's toxicity for infanticide

In Indian Mythology, Demon Pootana was, one of the chosen Poison Damsel, who tried to kill infant stage of Lord Krishna.

Damsel lady Pootna was sent by Mathura King Kansa for killing his infantile nephew lord Krishna, by breastfeeding laced with toxic opium, as she was the active secretor of opioids in her secretions- saliva, breast –milk, urine, sweat.

LETHAL LULLABIES:

Opium misuse to Infanticide:

Lullabies are soothing songs in rhymes, for making the infant sleep, by their babysitters, mostly.

But, in past, few babysitters used opium for inducing sleep to their infants, in care.

Poppy extract accompanied the human infant for more than 3 millenia.

Motives for its use included excessive crying, suspected pain, and diarrhea.

In antiquity, infantile sleeplessness was regarded as a disease.

When treatment with opium was recommended by Galen, Rhazes, and Avicenna, baby sedation made its way into early medical treatises and pediatric instructions.

Dabbing maternal nipples with bitter substances and drugging the infant with opium were used to hasten weaning.

A freerider of gum lancing, opiates joined the treatment of difficult teething in the 17th century.

Foundling hospitals and wet-nurses used them extensively.

With industrialization, private use was rampant among the working class.

In German-speaking countries, poppy extracts were administered in soups and pacifiers.

In English-speaking countries, proprietary drugs containing opium were marketed under names such as soothers, nostrums, anodynes, cordials, preservatives, and specifics and sold at the doorstep or in grocery stores.

Opium's toxicity for infants was common knowledge; thousands of cases of lethal intoxication had been reported from antiquity.

Obladen M. Lethal Lullabies: A History of Opium Use in Infants. J Hum Lact. 2016 Feb;32(1):75-85.

POISON DAMSELS DESCRIBED IN INDIAN MEDICO-LEGAL TREATISE:

In 1889, the mother of a 2 month old female child, left her child in verandah of her house, while she went to fetch water.

On returning she found the child sucking the finger of a woman who had come during her absence.

This woman on being asked, what she was doing hastily wiped her right hand in piece of rag and told the mother that she was giving the child some bread, a piece of which she showed in her left hand.

The woman than left, and the child soon commenced vomiting, and died within a few hours.

Opium was detected in the viscera of the child, and the rag on which accused woman wiped her finger was also found to bear stains of opium.

The bread which the accused held in the left hand contained no opium.

The mother wiped the mouth of the child, when it vomited with a piece of cloth which was also forwarded foe examination and in the stains on which opium was detected.

Citation: Lyon's Medical Jurisprudence for India With Illustra-
tive-Cases. Seventh Edition. Modes of Poisoning. p441.

THAT THE CHOSEN ONES WOULD BEEN ULTRA-RAPID METABOLIZER, CHIC;

Chic is a slang word used for complimenting beautiful attractive girl.

SCIENTIFIC HYPOTHESIS OF POISON DAMSELS:

That the chosen ones (विष कन्या) would been ultra-rapid metabolizer of opium.

As Poisoner might have multiple duplications of specific cytochrome P450 metabolizing opioids in their body.

On its chronic administration, instead of converting the normal 5% to 10% of codeine to morphine, they would convert nearly all into morphine, and excrete it all in their body fluids – saliva, breast milk, urine.

Opioid ultra-rapid metaboliser multiple duplications of specifics's cytochrome P450, Instead of converting the normal 5% to 10% of codeine prodrug to morphine.

Genetic polymorphisms of this Cyt P450 enzyme result in three phenotypes: poor metabolizer phenotype, extensive metabolizer phenotype, and ultrarapid metabolizer phenotype.

Ultrarapid metabolizers have duplication of the gene, resulting in increased enzymatic activity.

Poisoner would be converting nearly all of the toxic opioids.

Table 1. Case reports providing evidence on the impact of polymorphisms of metabolizing enzymes on the safety of codeine. Source: Eugenia Y. Pharmacogenomics and Opioid Analgesics: Clinical Implications. International Journal of Genomics Volume 2015, Article ID 368979, 8 pages

Author	Metabolizing enzyme	Polymorphism	Adverse event
Gasche et al., 2004	CYP2D6	CYP2D61 × 3, in a patient suffering from renal insufficiency and co-treated with CYP3A4 inhibitors	Life-threatening intoxication
Voronov et al., 2007	CYP2D6	CYP2D6 × 2	Apnoea and brain injury
Madadi et al., 2007	CYP2D6	CYP2D62A and CYP2D62 × 2	Death of the breastfed 13-day-old boy
Ciszkowski et al., 2009	CYP2D6	CYP2D61 × N	Death due to respiratory arrest
Kelly et al., 2012	CYP2D6	CYP2D61 × N	Two deaths, one case of severe respiratory depression

Y. Gasche, Y. Daali, M. Fathi et al., "Codeine intoxication associated with ultrarapid CYP2D6 metabolism," The New England Journal of Medicine, vol. 351, no. 27, pp. 2827–2831, 2004.

C. Ciszkowski, P. Madadi, M. S. Phillips, A. E. Lauwers, and G. Koren, "Codeine, ultrarapid-metabolism genotype, and post-operative death," The New England Journal of Medicine, vol. 361, no. 8, pp. 827–828, 2009.

P. Voronov, H. J. Przybylo, and N. Jagannathan, "Apnea in a child after oral codeine: a genetic variant—an ultra-rapid metabolizer," Paediatric Anaesthesia, vol. 17, no. 7, pp. 684–687, 2007.

P. Madadi, G. Koren, J. Cairns et al., "Safety of codeine during breastfeeding: fatal morphine poisoning in the breastfed neonate of a mother prescribed codeine," Canadian Family Physician, vol. 53, no. 1, pp. 33–35, 2007.

P. Madadi, C. J. D. Ross, M. R. Hayden et al., "Pharmacogenetics of neonatal opioid toxicity following maternal use of codeine during breastfeeding: a case-control study," Clinical Pharmacology and Therapeutics, vol. 85, no. 1, pp. 31–35, 2009.

L. E. Kelly, M. Rieder, J. van den Anker et al., "More codeine fatalities after tonsillectomy in North American children," Pediatrics, vol. 129, no. 5, pp. e1343–e1346, 2012.

Citation: Eugenia Y. Pharmacogenomics and Opioid Analgesics: Clinical Implications. International Journal of Genomics Volume 2015, Article ID 368979, 8 pages

A CASE OF DEATH OF
A BREAST FED BABY
13 DAYS AFTER BIRTH:

His mother was prescribed codeine as an analgesic after delivery.

Postmortem examination of stored breast milk samples showed morphine levels 4 times higher than expected. Upon genotyping, the mother was found to be heterozygous for a CYP2D6*2A allele and a CYP2D6*2 × 2 gene duplication.

Thus the mother had three functional CYP2D6 alleles and was classified as an ultrarapid metabolizer. The extra CYP2D6 enzyme resulted in increased O-demethylation of codeine to morphine, and consequently, very high concentrations of morphine were found in both the breast milk and in the blood from the child.

P. Madadi, G. Koren, J. Cairns et al., "Safety of codeine during breastfeeding: fatal morphine poisoning in the breastfed neonate of a mother prescribed codeine," Canadian Family Physician, vol. 53, no. 1, pp. 33–35, 2007.

CSI

Crime-Scene-Investigation (CSi) by Toxic-Detective Nurses.

Search for Toxic look- alike, Toxic- touch alike, Toxic sound-alike, Toxic taste- alike, Toxic smell-alike xenobiotics - on & around the victim, after checking scene safety as per WHO protocol: Dr. ABCDE (easy recall as name of some unknown toxic detective doctor)

This follows the general principles of life support given below: Dr-ABCDE

• D - DANGER - scene safety
• R - RESPONSE- call for help
• A – AIRWAY secured & maintain patency/ Antidote
• B – BREATHING support
• C – CIRCULATION maintain access
• D - DISABILITY/ Decontamination- Whole body
• E – EXPOSE THE PATIENT completely- to find poisonous bites/ stings
• F- Foley's catheterization for rapid excretion of toxic metabolites
• G-Gastric lavage for decontamination
• I- Isolation of patient & I-Intermittent rotation of Health Care provider to prevent further spread of toxicity to others (occupational hazards)

6-SENSES DEVELOPED FOR TOXIC-DETECTIVES

Simulation means imitation of a situation or process using the "5 Human Senses" for recognition:

1. See (using Eyes): Identify the poison/ toxin/ venomous animal/ toxic plant/ mushroom/ signs of specific intoxication.

2. Smell (using Nose): the noxious/fruity/aromatic/pungent odour of toxins.

3. Touch (using Hands): Simulated Victims /Snakes/ Spiders/ Scorpions look-alike rubber replicas for rapid & correct recognition.

4. Hear (using Ear): Sounds of venomous animals (Rattle snakes), moaning of victims of poisoning, Death rattle of laryngeal edema in need of urgent intubation.

5.Test (Never try to Taste with Tongue): Chemical Analysis of Poison.

6. Search 6Th Sense for Toxic- Detective is to utilize all the 5 senses together and using our knowledge & experience on common poisonings in India, in clinical correlation to specific toxidrome.

This is what we have developed in the" ISTOLS Toxidromal Approach" in managing Common Poisoning/ toxicity/ intoxication/ Envenomation with Xenobiotics. It's the latest term for any drug, poison, toxin venom causing injury to the humans by any route(oral/IV/IM/SC/Dermal) in any chemical form (Liquid, solid, gas)

Hope you all are able to understand & connect. Please share doubts, if any.

DURING CSI BY TOXIC DETECTIVE, NOTICE FOR:

- Toxic look- alike,
- Toxic sound- alike,
- Toxic taste- alike,
- Toxic smell-alike
- Toxic liquid-alike
- Toxic semisolid-paste-alike
- Toxic gas-alike
- Toxic face-alike
- Toxic colour-alike
- Toxic feel-alike
- Toxic- Taste alike

TOXIC-LOOK- ALIKE- POWDERS:

- White silky-like powder in nose = ketamine.
- White- crystalline powder in nose/pouch- bitter-taste= Cocaine
- Grey fine cement-like powder- mousy odour= Aluminium phosphide
- Black powder= Charcoal
- Bright orange/ red sindoor powder= Lead tetroxide
- Florescent yellow powder= Phosphorus

- Toxic-look- alike semisolid paste:
- Black paste in tongue/nose/hands with petrol like-smell= Toluene/ aromatic hydrocarbons (Boot polish)
- Black paste with burnt rope-like smell= Cannabis/marijuana
- Brown paste= Crude Opium extract

TOXIC-LOOK-ALIKE-LIQUIDS:

- White milk-like in small glass vial = Propofol
- White milk-like in medication glass bottle = Intralipid
- Bright blue/green liquid fluorescent to UV light = Antifreeze-ethylene glycol

TOXIC-SMELL-ALIKE

breath of victim:

- Mousy-like dead mouse= Phenylketonuria, Celphos-AlP
- Fishy odour: Zinc Phosphide
- Rotten Apples-like = Diabetic ketoacidosis, Alcohol – Red wines (as congeners in alcohol contains flavonoids derived from fermentation of fruits)
- Pear-alike smell (Acrid)= Chloral hydrate, paraldehyde
- Bitter almonds= Cyanide
- Garlic-like= Phosphorus, Al & Zn Phosphides
- Shoe-polish-like= Nitrobenzene
- Nail-polish-like smell= Acetone (diluent is nail polish is acetone)- Nail polish remover also contain acetone, Chloroform.
- Hand-rub like smell= isopropyl alcohol
- Pungent smell= Turpentine oil like= Organophosphates (diluent is turpentine oil)
- Rotten Eggs= H_2S
- Wintergreen oil-like smell (Iodex-like)= methyl salicylic acid
- Vinegar-like= Acetic acid
- Moth-balls like= Camphor, Naphthalene
- Hospital-like odor= Carbolic acid, Creosote

TOXIC-TASTE-
ALIKE LIQUIDS:

• Bitter = poisonous bitter bottle gourd juice. Neem- oil.
• All Alkaloids (amines derived from toxic plants) are bitter in taste- Opium, Digitalis, Quinine.
• Sour-like lemon= organic Acids, acetic acid, vinegar

TOXIC-LOOK-ALIKE-FACE:

• Dark grey face with dull appearance in severe hypotension: Aluminum phosphide. Dark grey face also develops in CKD & CLD patients on long term effects.
• Bluish lips & nails with gasping = Cyanosis= Opioids & Opiates
• Bright red Brick-like lips & blood= Cyanide (no cyanosis, contradictory to its sound-alike name=cyan)
• Yellow green= Jaundice due to Paracetamol, Mushroom liver toxicity
• Pale= Anaemic due to excessive internal/external bleeding in hemotoxic snake bite, warfarin anticoagulants toxicity.

• Toxic-spasms-alike focal seizure:
• Carpo-pedal spasm= Calcium channel blocker toxicity, hyperventilation
• Spasm of back muscles – opisthotonus- Tetanus

• Toxic-paralysis-alike Brain stroke: Botox toxicity in injected part of face.

TOXIC-SOUND-ALIKE

during auscultation of chest:

• Snoring / gasping = Respiratory failure- opioids & opiates.
• Musical= Bronchospasm – Beta blocker toxicity, anaphylaxis due to bee wasp sting
• Slurred voice- Alcohol toxicity, Brain stroke due to cocaine
• Silent chest- Apnoea/ severe bronchospasm
• Systolic Heart murmur- in Subacute bacterial endocarditis due to unhygienic injection of drugs of abuse.
• Moaning/ Crying- due to severe pain in corrosive burn outside/ inside, painful spasms in strychnine toxicity, conium toxicity.

TOXIC-LOOK

Eyes of victim:

• Half-closed-eyes-like myasthenia: Neurotoxic Cobra/Krait
• Closed eyes with dilated pupil: Opium, Alcohol
• Wide open eyes with constricted pupil: Cocaine, amphetamines, Ecstasy
• Uprolling of eyes with Seizures: Strychnine, Cocaine toxicity, Opiate withdrawal
• Fine lateral Nystagmus= Alcohol intoxication, Brain-stroke
• Vertical Nystagmus= PCP- phencyclidines

TOXIC-FEEL

alike touch the victim:

Hot & wet: Fever due to cellulitis- sepsis after injectable drugs of abuse

Hot & Dry: Anticholinergics overdose

Cold & Dry: Opioids (Cold turkey)

Cold & wet: Shock due to hypotension by AlP

TOXIC-FEEL-ALIKE

Radial-Pulse of the victim:

- Rapid & irregular= Atropine toxicity
- Slow & bounding= Organophosphates
- Rapid & thready= Aluminium phosphide
- Slow & Shallow= Opioids, Beta- blocker toxicity, Calcium channel Blocker toxicity, Digitalis toxicity

MODES OF CRIME

Investigated by Toxic detective

S-Suffering(Man-made) causing S- Sudden need of medical Skill (S-Skill is S added to kill) S-Supporting to -Save the life from the killing effort of accused by Indian Society of Life Support course:-

All S for easy recall:-
- S-Shooting- firearm
- S-Stabbing- knife
- S-Shocking- electric
- S-Sexual Assault
- S-Strangulation- hanging, ligature,

- S-Stupefying- Dhatura, Chloroform, GHB- for robbery/ rape/ ragging

- S-Sedating- Opioids, Opiates, Organophosphates (all O's for easy recall)

- S-Stimuation by all C's -Cocaine, Cannabis, Camphor

ACTIVATED CHARCOAL

Activated charcoal (antidote) - Powder binds Powder.

Charcoal: Black Powder binds White Powder.

Plants bind Plants- Charocal- plant product from burning wood, binds the toxins produced by plants- eg., Dhatura , Oleander, Digitalis, **Opium,** Calotropis

•Toxic Carbon products– CO, C2S, CCl4- Toxic gases.

Charcoal – Carcinogen.

•Activated Carbon charcoal (antidote) - Powder binds Powder.

•Charcoal hemoperfusion – detoxify blood from toxins circulating in systemic circulation

HEROIN

Q. Why its name Heroin?

Since in films, actor who is supported by heroine, becomes the winner in the end of the movie by showing heroic rescue. Similarly, it was marketed among soldiers as a drug, whose possession will bring out their heroic performance. Another fact related to its name is that the name heroin was chosen because it was to be a heroic cure for morphine addiction, as it was wrongly thought to be less abusive than morphine.

Q. What is traditional use of opioids in India & abroad?

Opium(अफीम) was the most popular painkiller for warriors in wars since its discovery. Opium was cultivated to get the opiates from its fruit juice. Rajputs were famous for fighting because they used to eat Opium just before going into battlefield. Its more of euphoria caused by opium, killing more enemies, forgetting their fears, and it acted as prophylactic painkiller for injuries caused in warfare.

Q. What are "Narcotics" in NDPS act?
Narcotic means sleep inducing agent. Legally It can be an opiate, opioids, cannabis, or cocaine(the very antithesis of a narcotic, since it is a stimulant).

Q. What is "Brown sugar" ?

Its slang term for Heroin, in crude form of brown crystals like sugar.

Q. What is term "death on the needle"?

Accidental deaths are relatively common from overdose especially among Intravenous abusers of Heroin.
Q. What paralytic infection is associated with the use of black
tar heroin?
Wound botulism (Clostridium botulinum) at injection site.

Q. What are opiates available?

Morphine, Heroine, codeine.

Q. What are opioids available?

Pethidine, Propoxyphene, Pentazocine, Fentanyl, Methadone,
Tramadol etc..

Q. How do opiates differ from opioids?

Opiates are specific substances derived from the opium poppy.
Opioids include all substances (both natural and synthetic)
that are capable of producing opium-like effects.

Q. Name three opioids that do not cause miosis.
Meperidine, propoxyphene, tramadol.

Q. Which opioid has cardiac fast sodium channel blocking properties?

Propoxyphene and its metabolite norpropoxyphene, both of
which cause QRS prolongation.

Q. What are clinical effects of opiate administration?

Analgesia, drowsiness, changes in mood (often euphoria)

Q. How do opioids exert effects?

Agonists of opioid receptors in the central and peripheral nervous systems and the GI tract.

Q. What are the cardiovascular effects of opioid overdose?
Hypotension and bradycardia.

Q. What are the dermatologic symptoms of opioid intoxication?
Flushing and pruritus (variably present).

Q. How are opioids metabolized and excreted?
Hepatic metabolism with renal excretion

Q. What are respiratory effects of opioid intoxication?
Respiratory depression, bronchospasm, and non-cardiogenic pulmonary edema. Fentanyl administration may be associated with chest wall rigidity.

Q. What is the cause of most opioid-related deaths?
Respiratory depression resulting in anoxia.

Q. How do opiates cause respiratory depression?
Direct effect on brainstem respiratory centers (through mu and delta receptors)

Q. What are the GI effects of opioid intoxication?
Nausea, vomiting, constipation

Q. How are opioids abused?
Depending on the specific substance, opioids can be insufflated,

injected, smoked, or taken orally.

Q. Why doctor should make MLC in every patient of suspected opioid poisoning?
MLC means informing police, so police can investigate on the site of crime & tell who gave, in what quantity, which substance by collecting evidence of vials used & taking statement form eye witnesses. If the patient has taken opioid by self for recreation, than he will be sent for de-addiction to prevent future episodes, as single dose can make the person dependent, if taken in high dose for getting euphoria. If the patient was poisoned by anyone else for stupefying in robbery or rape, than accused will be caught on time. If its accidental overdose by cancer patient, than raising MLC will prevent any allegation of medical negligence claims by patient's relatives later on, as Hospital has prepared MLC & sent samples on time for future defense to justify & detect drug levels & identify the drug consumed.

Q. What is the opioid toxidrome?
CNS and respiratory depression with miotic pupils.

Q. What is the general treatment of opioid poisoning?
Primarily supportive care. Respiratory depression will be the main concern. Naloxone may be used as a diagnostic tool or to avoid intubation.

Q. What is the opioid antagonist that is used to treat acute toxicity?
Naloxone, which competitively binds opioid receptors.

Q. Is there an antidote for opiate overdose?
Naloxone. It should be given slowly (0.4mg over a few min) and titrated with the return of spontaneous respiratory effort. As the half-life of naloxone is shorter than that of most opioids, the patient should be monitored for re-sedation or development of opioid-induced non- cardiogenic pulmonary edema,

typically manifesting within 4 hrs in people with normal renal function.

Q. What is the only drug approved during BLS (Basic life support) in opioid victims, which can be given even by non-medico?
According to AHA 2015 update, a bystander, family member or friend can administer Naloxone Intramuscular shot on arm or Naloxone intranasal spray in unconscious gasping victim due to suspected opioid overdose.

Q. What is the normal elimination half-life of naloxone?
30-60 min.
What medical condition results in prolongation of the elimination half-life of naloxone?
Renal failure

Q. Other than respiratory depression, what acute pulmonary complication is associated with opioid use?
Noncardiogenic pulmonary edema.

Q. What are the side effects of the fentanyl-based designer drugs?
Usual potency is greater than that of heroin, resulting in excessive sedation and death. Higher than usual doses of naloxone may be needed to reverse effects.

Q. What are "body packers" found at International airports?
Individuals who swallow wrapped packets of illicit drugs or insert such packets into body orifices. Most are asymptomatic but can have acute intoxications with rupture of the packets. If suspected, abdominal radiographs may be obtained, but packets present are not always radio-opaque. Consider whole bowel irrigation with polyethylene glycol (PEG-ELS). Surgical indications include bowel obstruction or intestinal perfor-

ation. Continuous infusion of naloxone may be indicated with rupture of heroin packets.

Q. What are "body stuffers"?
Individuals who swallow poorly wrapped or un-wrapped drugs, usually in an attempt to avoid police arrest. There is generally more likelihood of becoming symptomatic secondary to the exposure to the intestinal lumen. Because a person possessing heroine in his pockets, purse, bags or belongings is immediately arrested and get jailed for 10 yrs. There is death penalty for repeated offence.

Q. What is "small quantity" of different controlled drugs?
125mg of cocaine,
250mg of Heroin,
5gm of hashish ,charas, opium
500gm of ganja

Q. What are the signs of withdrawal?
CNS excitation (e.g., restlessness, agitation, anxiety, dysphoria), nausea, vomiting, abdominal cramps, diarrhea, piloerection, lacrimation, rhinorrhea, diaphoresis. AMS and fever are not associated with opioid withdrawal and those signs should prompt further diagnostic testing.

Q. Which medications have been used to alleviate opioid withdrawal symptoms?
Methadone, clonidine, buspirone.

Q. What percentage of the population lacks the ability to metabolize codeine to morphine?
Approximately 7% of the Caucasian population lacks the appropriate enzyme(CYP2D6).

Q. With opioid urine drug screens, what three opioids are reliably detected?

These screens detect morphine metabolites; therefore, only morphine, as well as heroin and codeine (both of which are metabolized to morphine), are detected by such screens. Other opioids (i.e., fentanyl, oxycodone, hydrocodone, meperidine, propoxyphene, hydromorphone, tramadol) may not be detected.

Q. What is prohibited under NDPS act?

NDPS Act, is an Act of the Parliament of India that prohibits a person to produce/manufacture/cultivate, possess, sell, purchase, transport, store, and/or consume any narcotic drug or psychotropic substance, except for therapeutic use by RMP at NDPS authorised Hospitals.

Q. it means any person possessing controlled drugs of addiction- morphine, heroin, LSD will be arrested by police on-spot?

Yes, police can arrest without warrant from magistrate, if any drug of addiction is found in possession of that person. Mostly, it happens at airports & rave parties in midnight.

Q. How will the cancer patient can possess "small quantity" morphine for his pain relief legally?

According to NDPS act, these drugs are permitted to be used for therapeutic purposes in good faith by medical personnels for treating patients. So, RMP prescribes morphine on his prescription for maximum duration7-10 days, Registered pharmacist can sale morphine at authorised pharmacy.

Q. What is importance of "small quantity" of Controlled drugs under NDPS act?

Lesser Punishment for illegal possession in "small quantity" is considered for "personal consumption", so if the arrested person claims that he is drug addict & has the Heroin drug for personal use only & he was not trying to sale it illegally commercially.

Q. What is NDPS act relevant for patients seeking opioids in emergency ?

NDPS act - Narcotics Drug addicts, if caught with the banned drug e.g., Heroin, can avoid imprisonment, if they are willing to reform by getting admitted to approved drug de-addiction psychiatric centre.

Q. Do drug addicts needs punishment by court or de-addiction for illegal possession of drug?
Courts are lenient towards drug-addicts on sympathetic grounds, as Law considers drug addicts as victims. So if arrested person proves that he is drug addict, and is willing to reform by promising that he wants to get cured of his addiction, than court sends them to de-addiction centre instead of prison jails.

Q. How arrested person can prove that he is drug addict, to save himself from imprisonment?
Arrested person seeks medicolegal examination by RMP, who will examine the arrested person, take blood & urine samples for detection of drugs of addiction. If found positive, they are sent to de-addiction instead of prison.

Q. What is medicolegal importance of 2014 amendment in NDPS act for Hospitals?
Parliament amended the NDPS Act to relax restrictions placed by the Act on Essential Narcotic Drugs (Morphine, Fentanyl and Methadone), making them more accessible for use in pain relief and palliative care. The Amendment also contained measures to improve treatment and care for people dependent on drugs, opened up the processing of opium and concentrated poppy straw to the private sector.

Q. What is medicolegal importance of 2014 amendment in NDPS act for Drug addict patients?

The Amendment also removed the NDPS Act's imposition of a mandatory death sentence in case of a repeat conviction for trafficking large quantities of drugs, giving courts the discretion to use the alternative sentence of 30 years imprisonment for repeat offences. However, the Amendment increased the punishment for "small quantity" offences from a maximum of 6 months to 1 year imprisonment. It strengthened provisions related to the forfeiture of property of persons arraigned on charges of drug trafficking.

OPIUM POPPY
FLOWER

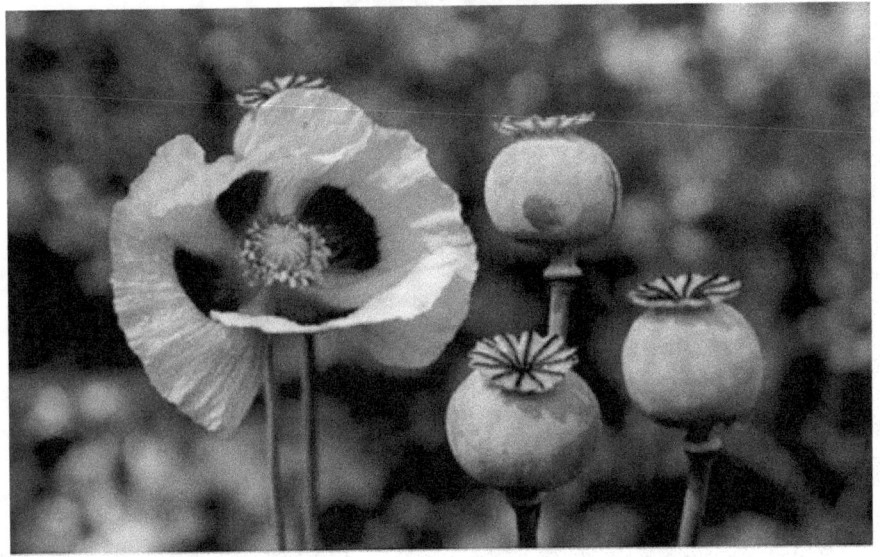

P-Poppy flower P-Petals in P-Pair of 4's - 4, 8, 12 ,
Petals are P-Papery thin & P-Pink in colour

89th Toxic Riddle in Rhymes

'This neat low gorse,

with golden boon,

Delights each sense,

is beauty, perfume;

And this gay ling, with

all its purple colours,

A man at leisure,

might admire for hours;

This green-fringed cup

moss has a scarlet tip;

Yields hundreds sap;

Its beads don't dip;

And then how fine enjoy

Holy herbage's sip!'

Guess this toxic convoy

Recurrent war to ship;

89

Riddle Analysis

P-Poisonous Poppy Plant identify - all P's for easy recall

All P's-Pinnate Leaves in Pairs of 2 oPPosite to each other,
Paper-thin Flower Petals in Pair of 4's,
Pods of Poppy, P- (पोस्त), Pain killers
P- Papaveraceae family – Pink /Purple flowers
P- Pain killers-oPium Poppies

P-पिला रंदे अफीम - Addiction
P-Poppy-पापी (Criminals) - illegal narcotics drug of abuse NDPS
P-Pop Singers abused it in past (Michael Jackson)
P-Pin P-Point P-Pupils
P-Paralysis of Breathing- Respiratory arrest- pH falls – Pulmonary

P-pH Peaks uP- Poppy Alkaloids- alkaline pH of gastric contents

P- Peela (पिला) flower seeds (पोस्त), P- Perpendicular Stems
P-Petals in Pairs of 4's- 4, 4x2 (8), 4x3 (12)
P- Prickly Poppy- Argemone Mexicana

'THIS NEAT LOW GORSE,

Gorse means a yellow-flowered shrub, typical look of opium crop, which looks like golden boon for its farmer, to earn good amount of money, on its sale.

POPPY FAMILY-PAPAVERACEAE– PINK /PURPLE/ PEELA FLOWERS

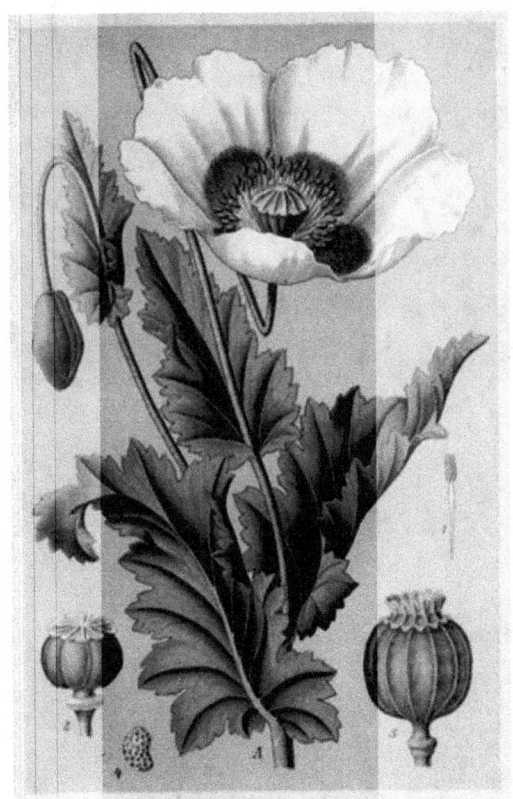

Pinnate Leaves & Papery thin Petals in flowers of Poppy

WITH GOLDEN BOON,

Opium's crude extract is golden brown in colour is equivalent worth to gold, as per weight.

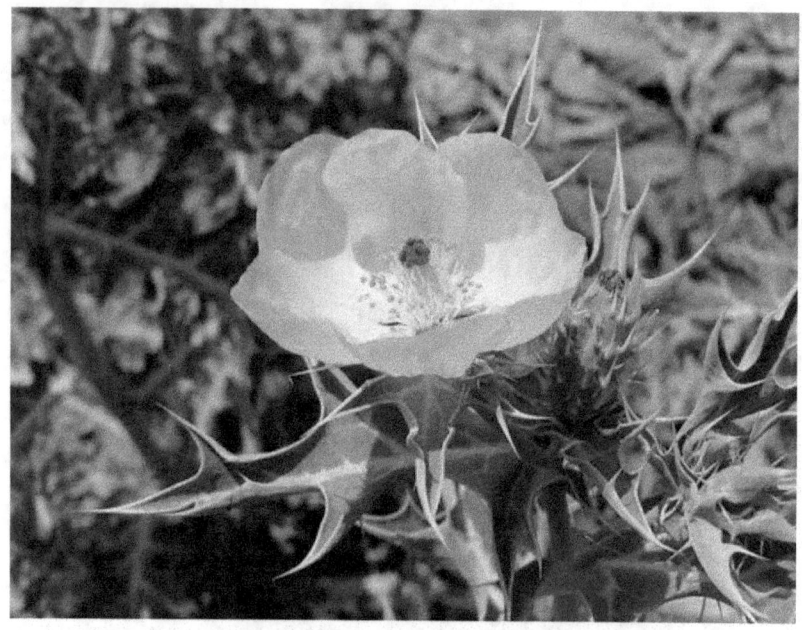

Peela cuP shaped flowers
with Prickly Pinnate
Leaves of Pickly Poppy Plant - Argemone Mexicana

DELIGHTS EACH
SENSE,

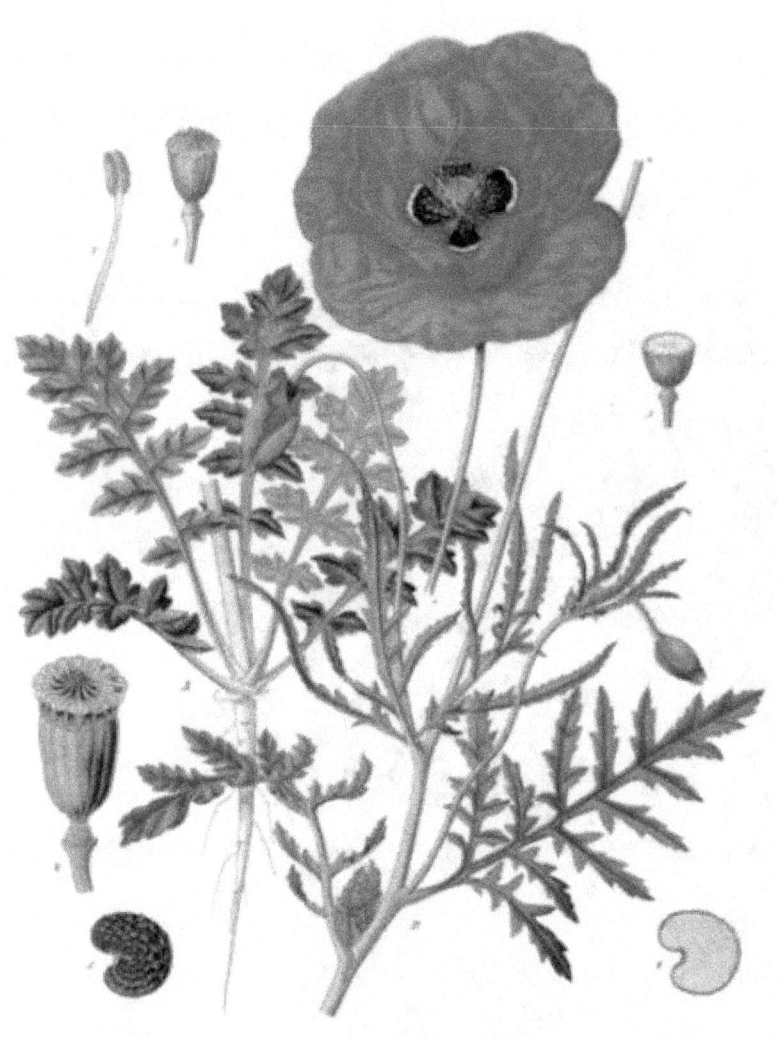

IS BEAUTY, PERFUME;

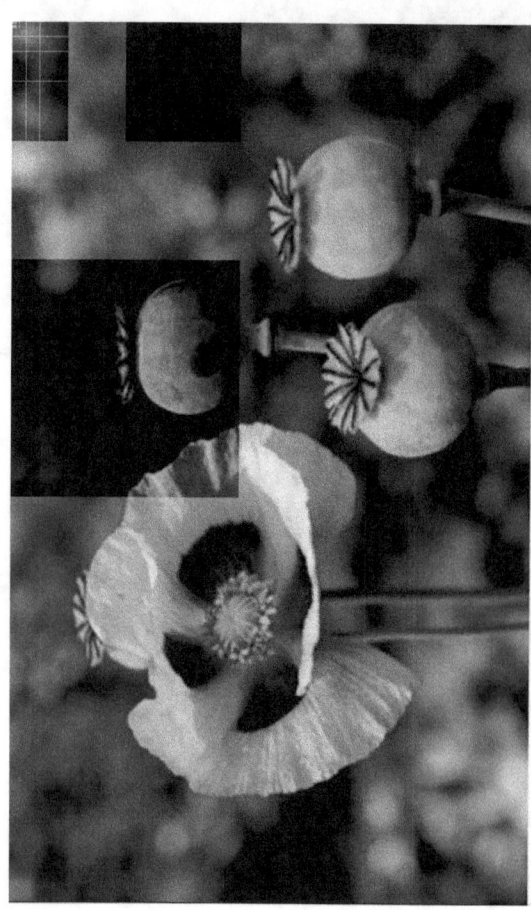

P-Poppy flower P-Petals in P-Pair of 4's - 4, 8, 12 , Petals are P-Papery thin & P-Pink in colour

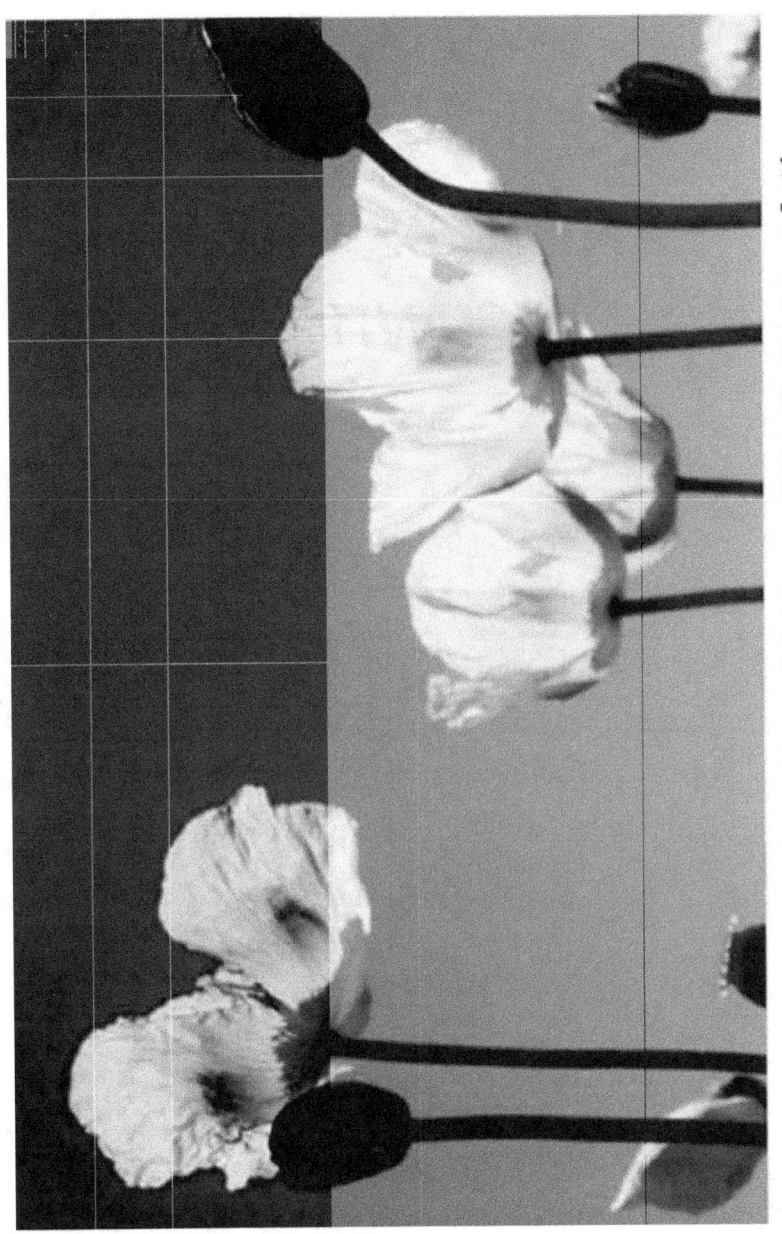

P-Papery thin P-Petals of P-Poppy in P-Pairs of 4's, transParent P-Pink in colour

AND THIS GAY
LING, WITH

ALL ITS PURPLE COLOURS,

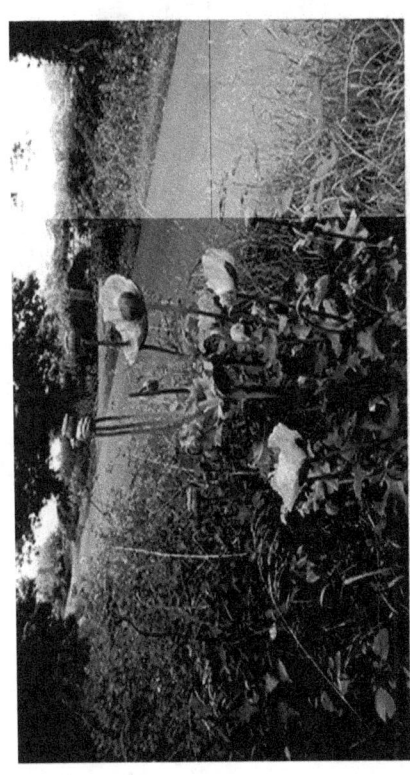

P-Pink cuP-shaped flowers with crePe P-Paper-thin P-Petals of P-Poppy plant with P-Pinnate leaves & P-Perpendicular stems uPward-facing, with P-Prickly hairs

A MAN AT LEISURE

Opium flowers are beautiful & attractive to sight, thus giving pleasure to the visitor, and opium poppy extract is abused to enjoy the leisure time, due to its pleasant feeling of well being & euphoria caused by opium.

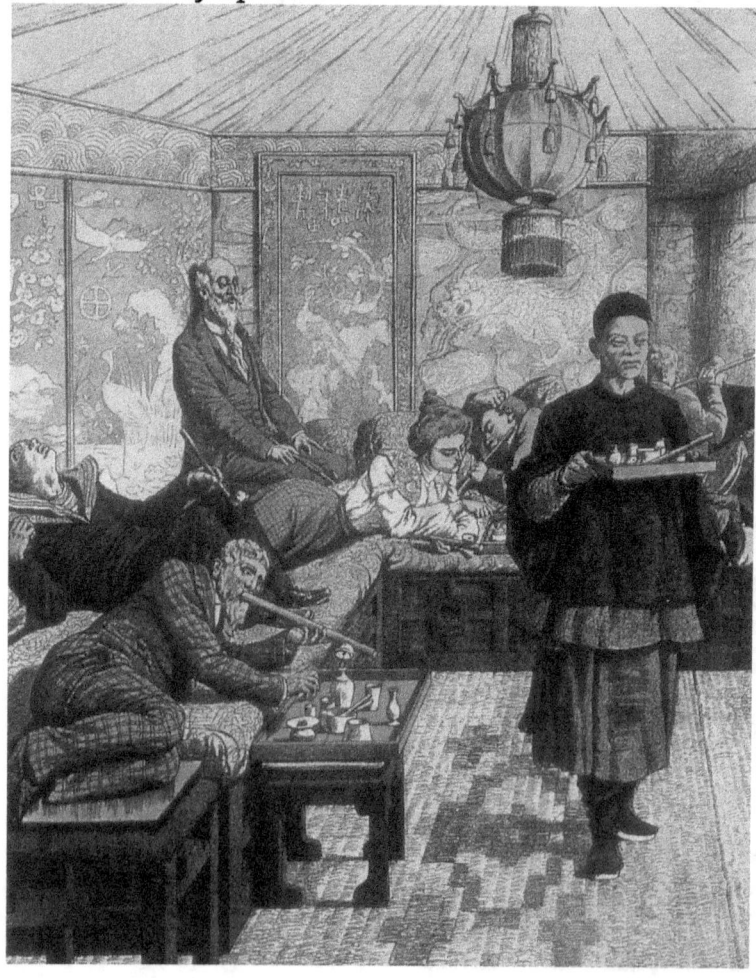

Political cartoon on Vishkanya

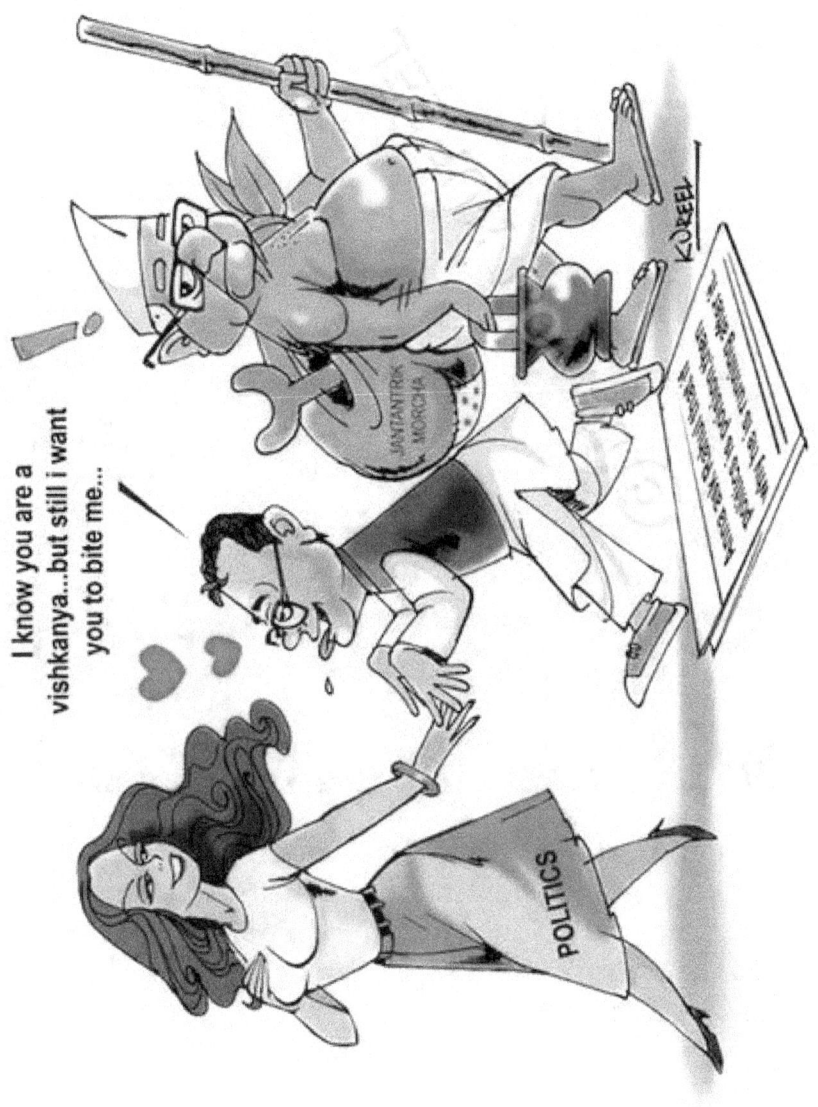

MIGHT ADMIRE
FOR HOURS

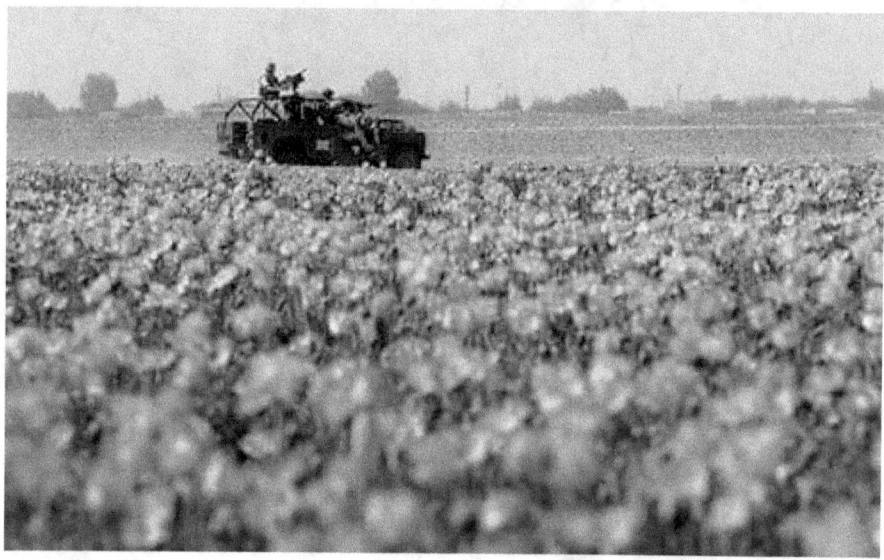

Opium farming has lead to wars, thus you can see a military tank, watching for preventing opium theft, by using weapons of mass destruction, as addicts craving for opium, attack in night, and rob the crop of opium, for satifying their urge or to smuggle opium & make easy money.

THIS GREEN-
FRINGED CUP

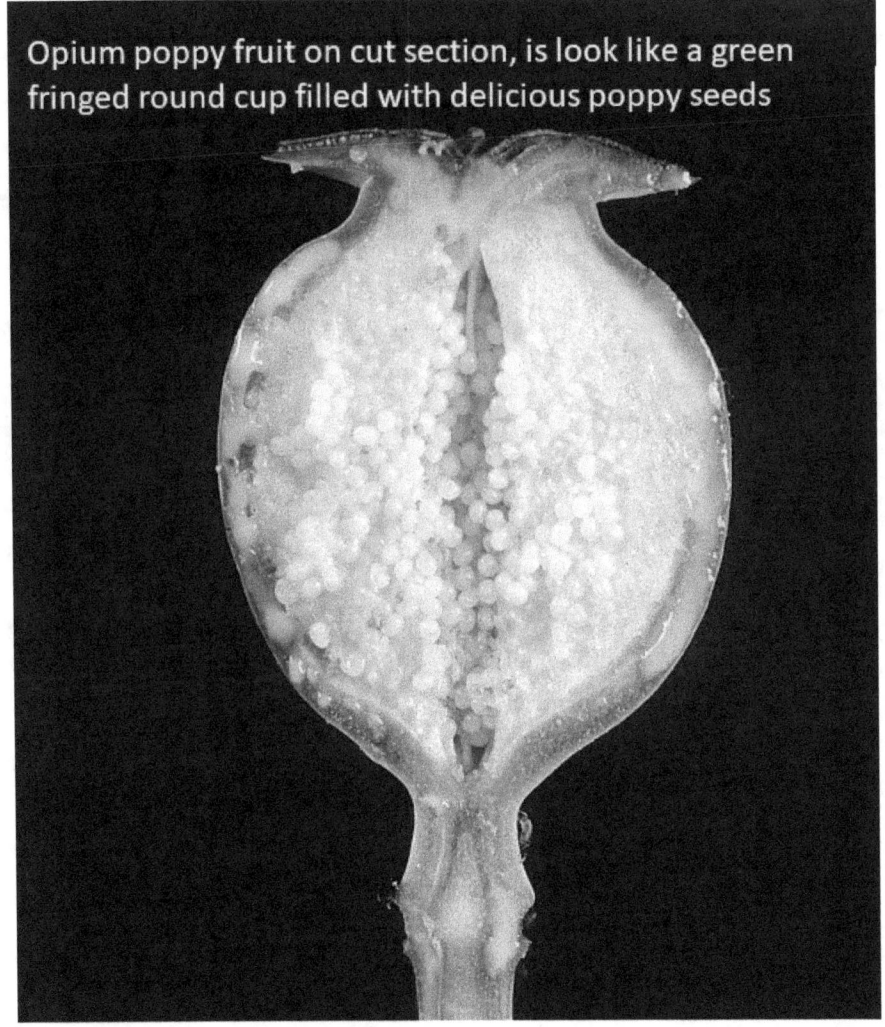

Opium poppy fruit on cut section, is look like a green fringed round cup filled with delicious poppy seeds

MOSS HAS A SCARLET TIP;

Marquis test: Bedside Colour test at crime scene

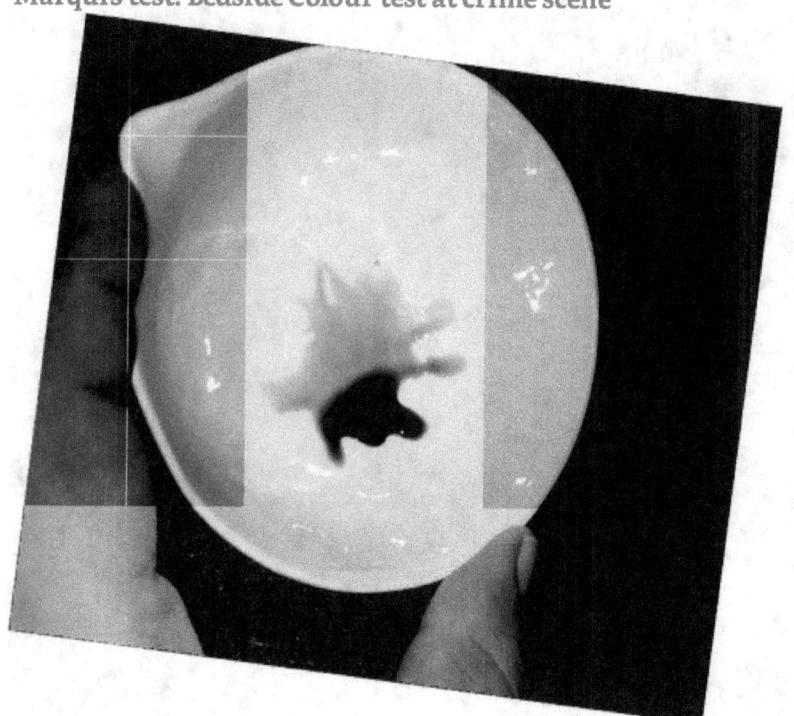

Add a mixture of 3 ml concentrated sulfuric acid and 3 drops of formalin to the gastric fluid.

A purple colour which gradually turns blue, indicates the presence of opium or its derivatives.

YIELDS HUNDREDS
SAP;

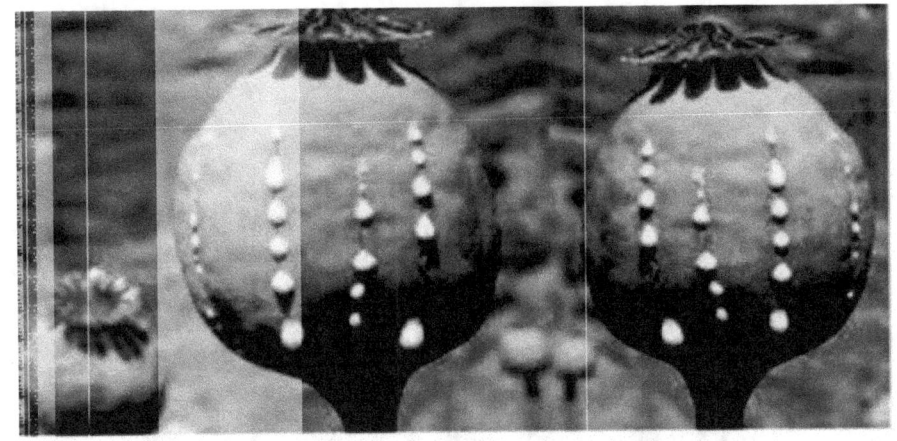

Poppy Pod with milky saP

ITS BEADS DON'T DIP;

Poppy seeds are just like beads which float on the drink made (Thandaai) during Holi festival

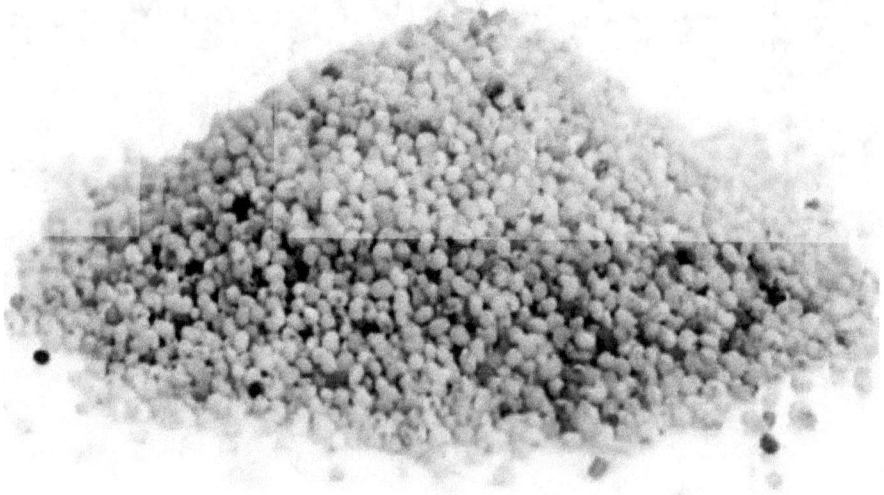

P-Poppy seeds P- Peela (पीला) flower seeds (पोस्त)

AND THEN HOW
FINE ENJOY

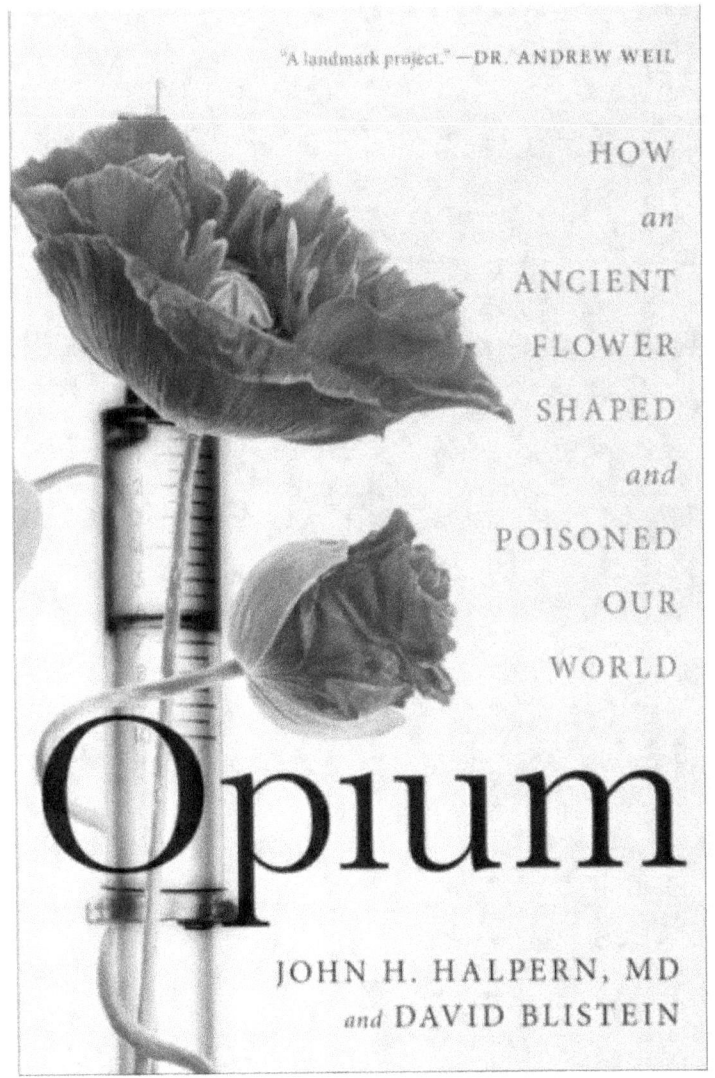

"A landmark project." —DR. ANDREW WEIL

HOW
an
ANCIENT
FLOWER
SHAPED
and
POISONED
OUR
WORLD

Opium

JOHN H. HALPERN, MD
and DAVID BLISTEIN

HOLY HERBAGE'S SIP!'

GUESS THIS TOXIC CONVOY

RECURRENT WAR
TO SHIP

Sea of Poppies & opium Wars from ships.

The Ibis trilogy is a work of historical fiction by Indian Author, Amitav Ghosh.

It deals with the trade of opium between India and China run by the East India Company and the trafficking of coolies to Mauritius.

It comprises Sea of Poppies (2008), River of Smoke (2011), and Flood of Fire (2015).

While some of the passengers of the Ibis reach their destination in Mauritius, others find themselves in Hong Kong and Canton and get caught up in events that lead to the First Opium War.

Sea of Poppies was shortlisted for the 2008 Booker Prize, while River of Smoke made it to the long list of the Man Asian Literary Prize in 2011.

https://en.wikipedia.org/wiki/Ibis_trilogy

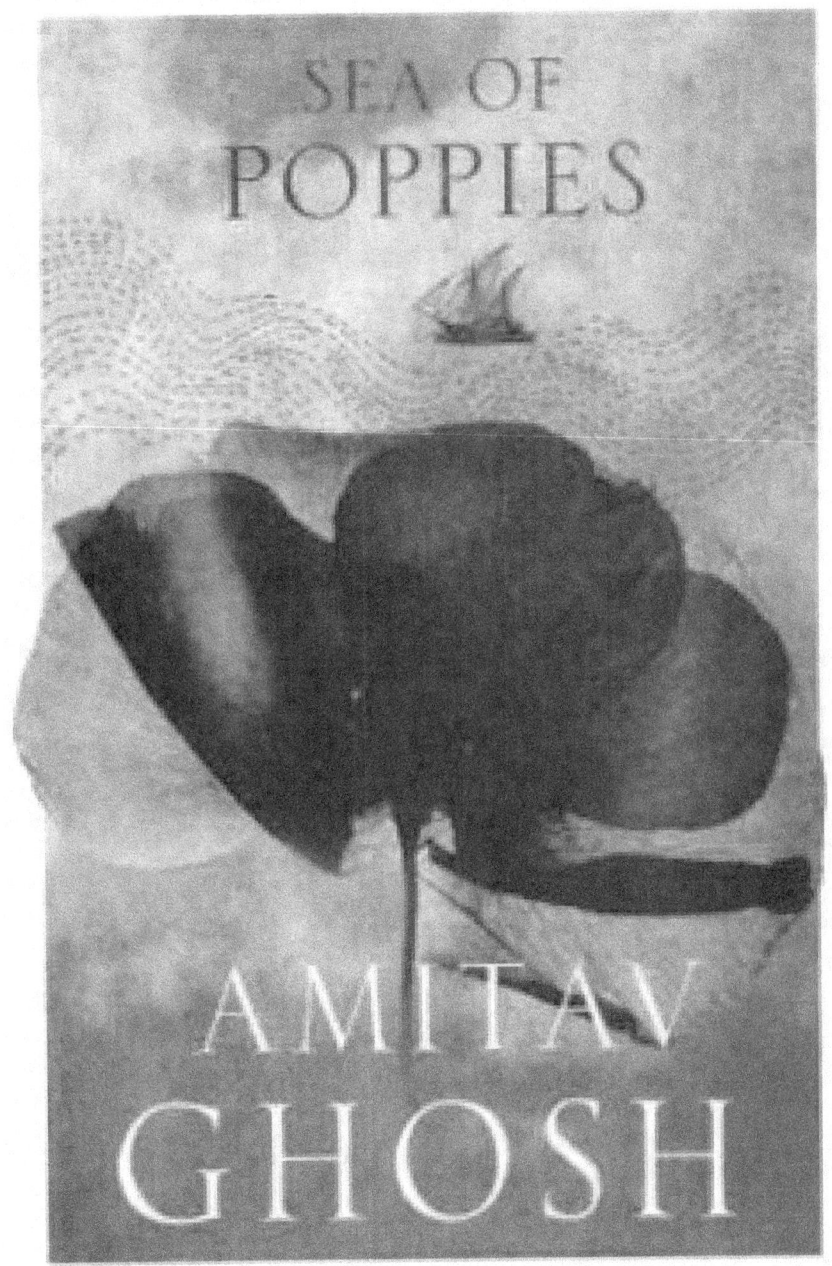

1ST HINT TO 89TH TOXIC RIDDLE:

For turning off its inflow tap

Its enforcement agency to trap

To prevent it's victims from crap;

Going into toxic irreversible nap;

So, Essential chemicals to scrap

Acetic anhydride in anyone's lap

To be notified of any use to map;

For Detergents to Printing inks in cap;

ACETIC ANHYDRIDE

Acetic anhydride is used commercially for preparing Detergents to Printing inks, has been found to be essential chemical for preparing heroin from morphine, and buying Acetic anhydride needs to be notified to the Drug Enforcement Administration (DEA) as per the Drug trafficking regulation;

Citation: Emsley J. Molecules at an Exhibition, Portraits of Intriguing Materials in Everyday Life. 1st Ed. Oxford Press. 2018.

Acetic Anhydride has also been declared precursor Chemical for use in the manufacture of illicit narcotic drugs and psychotropic substances.

Under NDPS Import policy, it is considered in the list as the 'Controlled Substances'.

This order issued under Section 9A of the NDPS Act, 1985 requires manufacturers, distributors, sellers, importers, exporters and consumers of specified controlled substances (Acetic Anhydride and others) to maintain records and file quarterly returns with the Narcotics Control Bureau.

Citation: Narcotic Drugs and Psychotropic Substances (Regulation of Controlled Substances Order) 2013, which came into force with effect from 26.03.2013.

2ND HINT TO 89TH RIDDLE

We all saw & read

Romeo & Juliet as

Shakespeare's creation;

Both didn't need

Any chemical assistance

To help them fall in love

Forming a love, relation.

But Juliet did however

Take this poison,

In undue resistance;

As part of her attempt to

Fool her family for duration;

Into thinking she had died,

For their love's existence;

A plan which backfired badly

in suspended animation;

Romeo found her

unresponsive on Bed;

Cold to touch, as dead,

So, for her nonexistence;

He took his own life, sad;

For meeting up together

In heaven's mansion

ROMEO AND JULIET: THE WAR TO LOVE

On analysis of the narration of Juliet's act in prose authored by Shakespeare, potion is most likely to be Opium (Morphine), as these plants are neurotoxic, and have the capacity to induce a coma with a respiration & heartbeat so slow it could be mistaken for death.

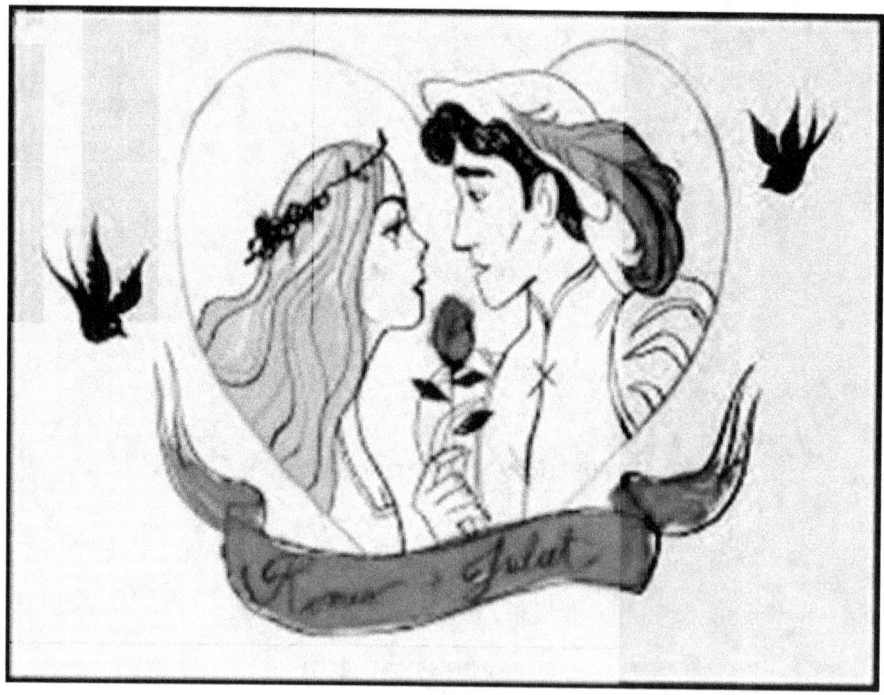

Opium makes its abuser to go in deep sleep of suspended animation; to be found her unresponsive on Bed; cold to touch, typical hypothermia suggestive of opioid toxidrome.

Sleeping draughts: Romeo and Juliet didn't need any chemical assistance to help them fall for each other.

Juliet did however take a mystery drug as part of her attempt to fool her family into thinking she had died, a plan which back-fired badly when Romeo found her and took his own life.

Juliet's Maid gave her the Opium extract saying:

"And in this borrowed likeness of shrunk death,

Thou shalt continue two and forty hours,

And then awake as from a pleasant sleep."

In the final act of Romeo and Juliet, Play's tragic heroine takes a potion to fake her own death and place her into a catatonic state.."

(Romeo and Juliet: Act 5, Scene 1).

Potion is most likely to be Opium (Morphine), as these plants are neurotoxic, and have the capacity to induce a coma with a respiration & heartbeat so slow it could be mistaken for death.

3RD HINT TO 89TH RIDDLE:

Its Den in Last,

On entry to past;

Displayed A warning

smoking is injurious to health

Illegal traders do sale it;

To increase their earnings

Buyer loose mind & wealth

It's smokes inhaled

in nose & lungs

Brings you near death

Risk Always hangs

How much damage it causes

Life endangered by it

And untimely pauses

Burns chain due to ashes

Smoker also turns into ash

Nail on ox may help in wash

Nothing will help

either money or cash

Thousands of deaths every year

Advice to its stop

may fall on deaf ear

They may hate to

heed or hear

Later on all brunt

we may bear

shared Amul in function

in cultural belief

Harms more, sought

& endanger lives

We hear but not

land ears or believe

Ends it in grave

damage then relieve

Harms may be more

than the advantage

Youth may be on wane

To die in early age

It is not piece of advice

Get help as simple device

Live life safe & simple way

Avoid it in total, as we say

2ND HINT TO 89
RIDDLE ANALYSIS

ITS DEN IN LAST,

ON ENTRY TO PAST;

DISPLAYED A WARNING

SMOKING IS INJURIOUS TO HEALTH

ILLEGAL TRADERS DO SALE IT;

TO INCREASE THEIR EARNINGS

BUYER LOOSE MIND & WEALTH

IT'S SMOKES INHALED

IN NOSE & LUNGS

BRINGS YOU NEAR DEATH

RISK ALWAYS HANGS

HOW MUCH DAMAGE IT CAUSES

LIFE ENDANGERED BY IT

AND UNTIMELY PAUSES

BURNS CHAIN
DUE TO ASHES

Chain Due= Chandu

चंडू (Chandu) Smoked from of opium in special elongated pipe prevalent in China & India.

Chandu is a Malay word which means energetic

चंडू = Chandu= Zandu

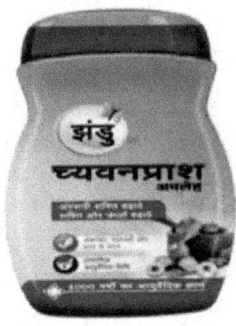

Figure 3. Zandu word derived from chandu but doesn't contain any opioids

SMOKER ALSO TURNS INTO ASH

NAIL ON OX MAY
HELP IN WASH

Nail On Ox= Naloxone

Opioid toxicity & its antidote Naloxone

Q. What is goal of Naloxone in Opioid Overdose?

The goal of the administration of naloxone is to restore adequate ventilation, rather than to reverse all the effects of the opioid and potentially precipitate withdrawal. Naloxone can be administered   intravenously, intramuscularly, and subcutaneously, but in patients who are in respiratory arrest, naloxone is often administered nasally (perhaps by a trained bystander) at a dose of 2 mg or 4 mg, which can be repeated, if needed.

Q. What are some of the features of opioid-induced noncardiogenic pulmonary edema?

Noncardiogenic pulmonary edema occurs as a complication of opioid   overdose in approximately 0.8 to 2.4% of cases. The majority of   patients who have noncardiogenic pulmonary edema related to opioid   overdose have respiratory symptoms immediately after overdose, but   the symptoms may be delayed up to 4 hours. Treatment consists of   supportive therapy with supplemental oxygen; mechanical ventilation   is required in approximately one third of patients. Symptoms resolve   within 24 to 48 hours in the majority of patients.

Q. What physician practices may help in preventing opioid overdose?
The prevention of opioid overdoses requires a multifaceted approach.   Primary prevention of opioid-use disorder involves limiting a   patient's exposure to prescription opioids, starting with the first   encounter. Patients for whom opioid prescriptions are considered   should be assessed with the use of a prescription-monitoring program.   If opioids are prescribed, a defined treatment plan should be discussed with the patient. Both the dose and the duration of the   first opioid prescription should be limited, since the probability of   prolonged opioid use increases linearly with the number of days for which the drug is initially supplied. Patients who already use   opioids should be considered to be at risk for possible overdose, and   secondary prevention

efforts could be initiated. When patients   receive opioids in the emergency department, they could be offered   kits that contain naloxone, an opioid antagonist. Patients' friends   and family could also be offered kits and training in overdose   recognition, so that they can administer naloxone if needed.

Q: What are some of the recommended emergency department measures for the management of opioid overdose?

A: Reversal is only the first step in the management of opioid overdose in the emergency department. In ER, patients who are   resuscitated after an opioid overdose are offered an evaluation for   substance-use disorder before discharge, with the goal of helping   them to connect with inpatient and outpatient resources for long-term   treatment of addiction. Evidence shows that inpatient detoxification   programs are of limited value and the most effective approach is   long-term opioid-agonist therapy with methadone or buprenorphine,   which increases treatment retention and reduces ongoing opioid use,   health care costs, and mortality. Initiation of addiction treatment   with buprenorphine or methadone in the general hospital or emergency department is a strategy that results in higher rates of treatment retention than do detoxification programs or referrals to community treatment. Although psychosocial services should be made available to all patients, medication alone effectively reduces ongoing opioid use.

Q: What factors contribute to limited access to or use of opioid-agonist therapy for opioid addiction?

A: Access to opioid-agonist therapy remains limited. Only 1% of   specialists in emergency medicine have waivers that allow them to   prescribe buprenorphine, and half the counties in the United States   do not have a single specialist who can prescribe buprenorphine.

Qualitative studies that included people who had been incarcerated showed that fear of forced withdrawal led them to opt against   opioid-agonist therapy. In addition, the standard practice of forced   withdrawal of opioid-agonist therapy at the time of incarceration   results in lower treatment retention in the community after release.   A major barrier to expanding the use of opioid-agonist therapy is   stigma perpetuated by the widely held misperception that these   medications "replace one addiction with another." Despite the vast   amount of data supporting the use of opioid-agonist therapy,   physicians are not immune to this stigma. The prevailing societal   view that people with addiction have "brought upon themselves the   suffering they deserve" may also affect physicians and contribute to   the low frequency of offering buprenorphine treatment.

NOTHING WILL HELP

EITHER MONEY
OR CASH

THOUSANDS OF
DEATHS EVERY YEAR

ADVICE TO ITS STOP

MAY FALL ON DEAF EAR

THEY MAY HATE TO

HEED OR HEAR

LATER ON ALL BRUNT

WE MAY BEAR

SHARED AMUL
IN FUNCTION

अमल = मलरहित (means without any dirt)

That's how this name got adopted into *AMUL*, for the popular indian brand of milk & butter, as its safe to eat, without any dirt.

AMUL= Anand Mill United Limited

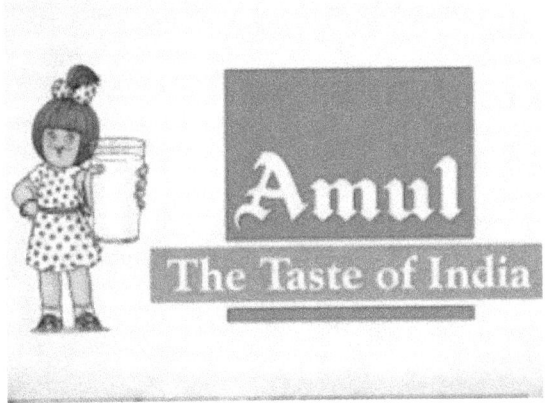

Figure 4. Amul products doesn't contain any opioids. Its just co-incidence, that the names are similar

Amul products doesn't contain any opioids

During Medieval period indian Rajput warriors used to eat opium together, is the most inviolable pledge, and an agreement gratified by this ceremony is stronger than any adjuration.

Umul Liya ?

Have you had your opiate ?

DR VIVEKANSHU VERMA FIST

Umul kao
" Take your opiate."

IN CULTURAL BELIEF

HARMS MORE, SOUGHT

& ENDANGER LIVES

WE HEAR BUT NOT

LAND EARS OR BELIEVE

ENDS IT IN GRAVE

DAMAGE THEN RELIEVE

HARMS MAY BE MORE

THAN THE ADVANTAGE

YOUTH MAY BE ON WANE

TO DIE IN EARLY AGE

IT IS NOT PIECE OF ADVICE

GET HELP AS SIMPLE DEVICE

LIVE LIFE SAFE & SIMPLE WAY

AVOID IT IN TOTAL, AS WE SAY

CHAIN DUE= CHANDOO/ CHANDU (HOMONYMOUS WORDS)

(चंडू Smoked from of opium in special elongated pipe prevalent in China & India)

Its consumption delight the senses to its abuser, especially when its smoked per-fume with elongated pipes in China (opium pills used for smoking were named as Chan-du).

The term chandu is believed to originate from the Malay language.

Citation: Carl A. Trocki (1999). Opium, Empire and the Global Political Economy: A Study of the Asian Opium Trade, 1750-1950. Psychology Press

AMUL= UMUL (HOMONYMOUS WORDS)

अमल is the liquid form of opium shared among Rajput community, still now, in hidden manner.

अमल = मलरहित (means without any dirt) Literally it meant bonding without any bad intention or ill feelings or thoughts to harm each other.

That's how this name got adopted into *Amul*, for the popular indian brand of milk & butter, as its safe to eat, without any dirt.

On any family occasion of marriage or childbirth, they celebrate by saying Umul, as it gives pleasure & increases bonding to associates.

This tradition came from past phase of recurrent wars, in which the warriors consumed opium and went to war.

As its strong pain reliever, so the painful stabbing wounds, will not be that painful to stop the warrior fighting till fatal injury to him.

The vice of opium -eating is a very ancient practice in India, especially among the Rajpoots.

Todd, who wrote Rajputana's history, frequently alludes to it in his Rajasthan.

The date of the introduction of opium into India cannot be traced.

The act of eating opium together was the form by which rival clans became reconciled, and personal friendships were declared.

" Umul lar kana,"to eat opium together, is the most inviolable pledge, and an agreement gratified by this ceremony is stronger than any adjuration.

If a Rajpoot pays a visit, the first question is

Umul hya ? Have you had your opiate ?

Umul kao " Take your opiate."

On a birth-day, when all the chiefs convene to congratulate their brother on another "knot to his years," the large cup is brought forth, a lump of opium is put therein, upon which water is poured, and by the aid of a stick, a solution is made, to which each helps his neighbour, not with a glass, but with the hollow of his hand held to his mouth.

A Rajpoot is fit for nothing without his umul.

(Chevers Manual of Medical Jurisprudence for India, 1870)

Roughly 450,000 people died as a result of drug use in 2015.

Of those deaths, about 160 thousands were directly associated with drug use disorders and about 118 thousands with opioid use disorders.

(Citation: WHO factsheet on opioid overdose)

Nail-on-ox = Naloxone (Antidote to Opium)

Until the invention of Naloxone & naltrexone, as the pharmacological antidote to opium, Atropa was actually used to antagonise the action of opium, and vice versa.

Reversal of the size of the pupil, was thought as the sign of recovery, although it was later found to be misleading finding.

Agitation in Atropa toxicity was treated with opium, to sedate the patient, but had high risk of aspiration & sudden respiratory arrest. (Chevers Manual of Medical Jurisprudence for India, 1870)

18TH TOXIC MURDER NARRATED IN RHYMES;

Riddles during Terror of Corona times;

By Toxic Detective solving Crimes;

On Indian Society of Toxicology (IST)'s Paradigms;

Intentional food Poisoning for hostile purposes,
misusing Blind Faith of religious race;

The accused was working as an elderly priest
doing worship in common space;

60yrs old Victim was a member of the Managing
Committee of that holy place;

60yr old Accused had a grudge with that senior
citizen for public disgrace;

During Argument Over ownership of managing
committee face to face;

And victim made several complaints in past,
against accused, to worse the case;

For his removal from the post of priest, and reinstate

him on his place;

One day, in the early hours of the day, searching
to victimise his chase;

Accused gave a morsel of sacred food, in pleasant
mood, and poker face, for Almighty God's sake;

Sacred food offered at religious places, no pious
follower of the faith, would refuse or misplace;

Masking poison's bitter taste, laced in sweetest recipe,
to make it inconspicuous to efface,

After some time, Victim felt sick, giddy, drowsy
and his heart began to sink, in pace;

Other holy men co-workers, took notice of his difficulty
in breathing, imbalance & sleepy, interlace;

Inspite of the medical aid he could not survive,
as his arterial pH & vital gases debased;

And died about 4 hrs after administration of toxin,
displaying blue lips & nails, like carcase;

Court found that accused had a motive to commit
murder & its not food poisoning, just by mistake;

And he did it with an intention to kill the deceased,
with cold blooded rivalry to embrace;

Accused was convicted for culpable homicide
amounting to murder, misusing trust, in case;

For murder of the victim in preplanned manner,
to take the revenge for public disgrace;

With clear motive & intention to kill the victim,
at holy site with toxic *coup de grace*;

By misusing fatal poison in fatal dose, for lethal
outcome, without any remorse, with poker face;

Guess the toxin & the real-life-case discussed to *retrace:*

HINT: HOLY FOOD: PRASAAD:

Opium killer

It became the landmark case in Crime History for setting up guidelines of exceptions, which actually helped later sentenced criminals with capital punishment (not this case accused), to claim for relaxation to not get hanged, and commute the life threatening status, with petition of appeal to sentence of life imprisonment; on grounds of elderly age, gender, pregnancy, as special case to get exempted from getting hanged till death.

1.   Supreme court decision in case of Balwant singh Vs State of Punjab; AIR 1976 SC 230: 1976 Cr LJ 291: (1976)1 SCC 425. https://indiankanoon.org/doc/1981063/

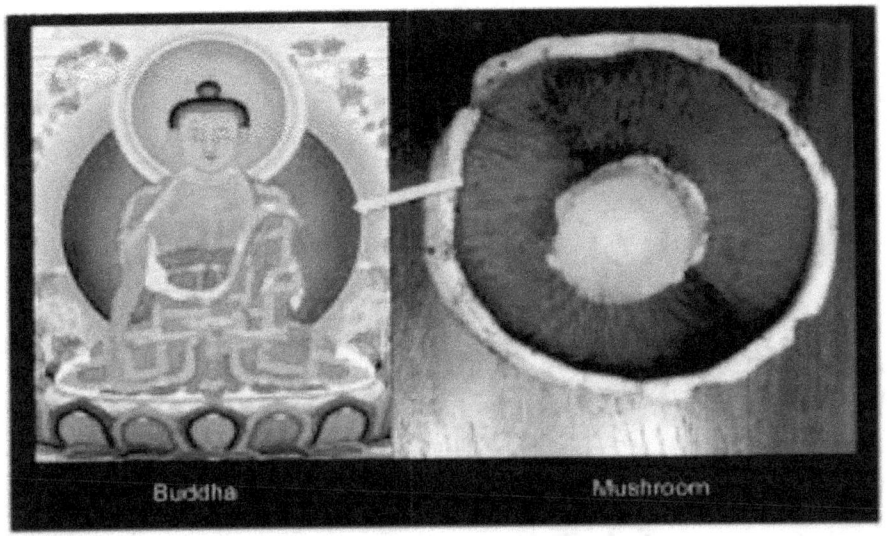

Buddha — Mushroom

Mushroom Toxicity

483 years Before Christ, Poisoning Victim was an Aged Superior Being; Lord Buddha.

Toxic dysentery resulted in decline of health and death later.

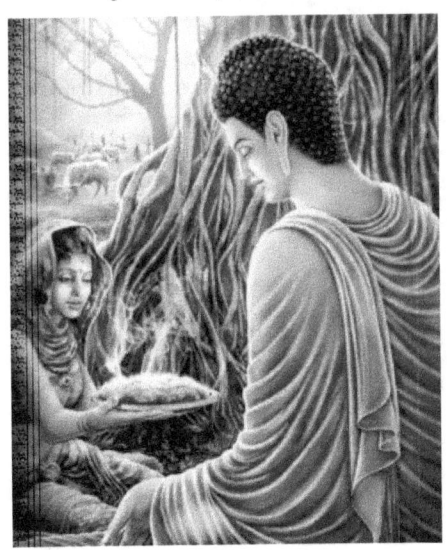

POISONOUS ROBES
= जहरीली ख़िलअत

King's Poisoning Device as Robes of Honour.

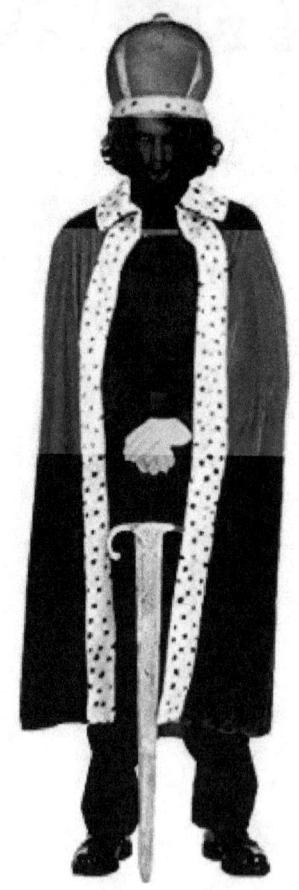

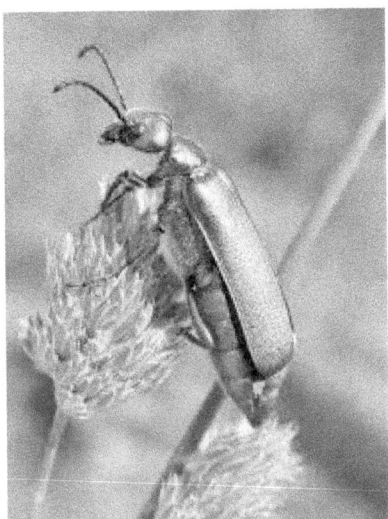

A Rathore prince, was thus killed to death by a robe of honor presented to him by Aurangzeb in 1700 AD.

The Queen of Ganore killed Khan, by Robe in 1723, jumped in the Narmada to save her Honour

Robe cloth were thoroughly impregnated with the Cantharidin (Spanish Fly= Green Beetle) of that very powerful vesicant, which would result in extensive chemical burn, and painful death due to sepsis.

Cantharidin is popular aphrodisiac (A myth), as it causes priapism (A fact)

CONTRIBUTORS

1. Dr Yatin Mehta, Chairman, Anaesthesia, Critical Care, Emergency & Trauma care, Medanta-The Medicity, Gurugram
2. Dr P Venugopalan, Director, Emergency & Trauma care, MIMS, Calicut
3. Mr Santosh Kumar Verma, Senior Advocate, Rajasthan High Court
4. Dr Tariq Ali, Director, Critical Care, Medanta-The Medicity, Gurugram
5. Dr Praveen Aggarwal, Professor & Head, Department of Emergency Medicine, AIIMS, New Delhi
6. Dr Venkat Raghav, Professor & HOD, Forensic Medicine & toxicology, Bangalore Medical College, Bengaluru.
7. Dr Ajay Gangele, Professor, Forensic Medicine & Toxicology, DY Patil Medical college, Pune
8. Dr Krishnadutt Chavali, Professor, Forensic Medicine & Toxicology, AIIMS, Raipur
9. Dr SK Singhal, Professor &HOD, Forensic Medicine & Toxicology, Ananta Institute of Medical sciences and research center, Rajsamand (Rajasthan).
10. Dr Dhruv Chaudhary, Senior Professor & Head, Pulmonary & Critical Care Medicine, PGIMS, Rohtak
11. Dr Tejas Prajapati, Consultant Toxicologist, AMC MET Medical College, Ahmedabad, Gujarat
12. Dr Karen Harshita, Senior Resident, Forensic Medicine & Toxicology, Bangalore medical College and research institute, Bangalore
13. Dr Ajith Antony Senior Resident, Forensic Medicine & Toxicology, Goa
14. Dr Lishu Chaure, Senior Resident, Palamu Medical College,

Palamu Jharkhand.

15. Dr Somashekar Chandren, Assistant professor Forensic Medicine & Toxicology, AIMS, B G Nagara, Mandya, Karnataka

16. Dr Latif Johnson, Assistant professor, Forensic Medicine & Toxicology, Christain Medical College, Vellore

17. Dr Arjit Dey, Senior Resident, Forensic Medicine & Toxicology, AIIMS, Delhi

18. Dr Kashif Ali, Senior Resident, Forensic Medicine & Toxicology, Jawaharlal Nehru Medical College, AMU, Aligarh (UP)

19. Dr. Sweta H Patel, Assistant Professor, Forensic Medicine & Toxicology, Pramukhswami Medical College, Karamsad. Dist. Anand, Gujarat.

20. Dr Suman K. Charawati, Scientist, Forensic Science Lab, Assam

21. Dr Walter Waz, Professor, Forensic Medicine & Toxicology, Mumbai

22. Dr Vidusha Vijay, Forensic Medicine & Toxicology Consultant, Columbia Asia Hospital Bangalore.

23. R. R. Rajitha, Emergency Nursing officer, King Faisal Hospital, Riyadh, Saudi Arabia

Poison Damsels as Biological Weapons in ancient warfare & its Pharmacogenomics: Thousands of cases of lethal intoxication had been reported from antiquity.
In 320 BC, King Chandragupta attempted to kill Alexander the Great, by sending Poison Damsels, as concubine of the king. Since past, these chosen females, who were found to be hyper secretors of toxins fed to them, got trained, for killing their royal victims tactfully. Opium was one of the most common toxins given for killing precious royal princes mostly for infanticide.
In Indian Mythology, Demon Pootana was, one of the Poison Damsel, who tried to kill infantile Lord Krishna. As the chosen ones were ultra-rapid metabolizer of opium. These Poisoners might have multiple duplications of specific cytochrome P450 metabolizing opioids in their body.

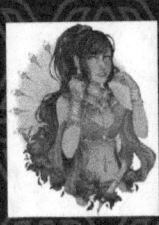

Discovering these toxicological mysteries, hidden in our ancient mythology, with logical hypothesis on scientific basis, decoding myths, is the clue to solve these toxic riddles

Vivekanshu Verma
Vijay Vasudev Pillay
Shiv Rattan Kochar
Prateek Rastogi

ACKNOWLEDGEMENT

We are grateful to the whole team of Amazon Kindle Publications Pvt Ltd, Editor & Production Manager & Book designer team of the Amazon publishers, USA who helped & guided with their team members for all their support to the work in this project and make this book project a success.

We are thankful to Dr Gopalan Sir, Mr Kevin and the whole team of Amrita Simulation Lab, AIMS, Kochi, who helped in the Indian Society of Toxicology Life Support (ISTOLS) simulation training to make it useful for nurses & doctors.

We are thankful to members of our Critical Care Department at Medanta- the Medicity, who all morally supported us to make this edition possible, and gave a nurturing environment, in compiling the critical care in toxicological emergencies.

We thank our Emergency team - Dr Devendra Richhariya, Dr Sudhir Singh Pawaiya, Dr Sunil Dubey, Dr Hashim Mozzan, Dr Sharad Manar, Dr Shashank Chauhan, Dr Vikram Pattanaik, Dr Mansih Sachdeva, Dr Shailendra Arya, Dr Neeraj Sharma, Dr Raman Mathur, Dr Joe keerti, Dr Bala Prakash, Dr Tinu Saseendran, Dr Jidhin Janardan, Dr Anukriti Jain, Dr Dilip Patel, Dr Rosika Chawla, Dr Sabina, Dr Parvathy, Dr Divya, Dr Ajay GS, Dr Narsh, Dr Ekum and others, who supported us in academic activities.

We are especially grateful for the contributions from our Emergency Nursing officers, Medanta- the Medicity, Sector 38, Gurugram, including : Mr Sumer Singh, Mr Thomas Chacko, Mr Jinu Johnson, Mr Amir Khan, Mr Peney Abraham, Mr Retheesh K. K., Ms Sunita, Ms Manisha, Ms Sapna Bhardwaj, Ms Reetu , Ms Priyanka, Ms Manju, Ms Richa Thakur, Ms Vandana Kumari, Romy, Ms Bhawana, Ms Priya, Ms Shraddha, Ms Prabhjot Kaur Deol, Ms Ritika Rana, Ms Athira Babu, Ms Amandeep, Ms Komal Dubey, Ms Shilpa Rana, Ms Chaynika, Ms Priyanka Patidar, Ms Divya, Ms Jesslin Jose, Ms Merlin Thomas, Rohitash, Ritu Raj, Ms Alfy Mariya , Kashi, Mr. Paneer, Ms Jisha, Ms Nisha, Ms Satpal, Sayed, Ms Anchal Kumari, Ms Rajni, Ms Sapna Kumari, Ms Jeenamol, Ms Seema,Ms Anjali, Ms Nancy, Ms Sakshi, Ms Shiva Rajpoot, Mohit Kumar Sharma, Susheel Tiwari, Vijay Kumar, Sijo, Ramniwas Bissu, Ahamad Hussain, Mukesh Kumar, Rajiv Fateh Masih, Upendra Kumar, Ms Neelam, Nadeem, Manoj Kumar, Ankush, Madhvan, Mohamed Mahadeer , Ms Varsha, Solen, Pardeep Nar , Neeraj, Kuldeep Singh, Ms Mansi, Ms Manpreet Kaur , Ms Preeti, Ms Ritika, Ms Priyanka, Ms Gayatri Lahre.

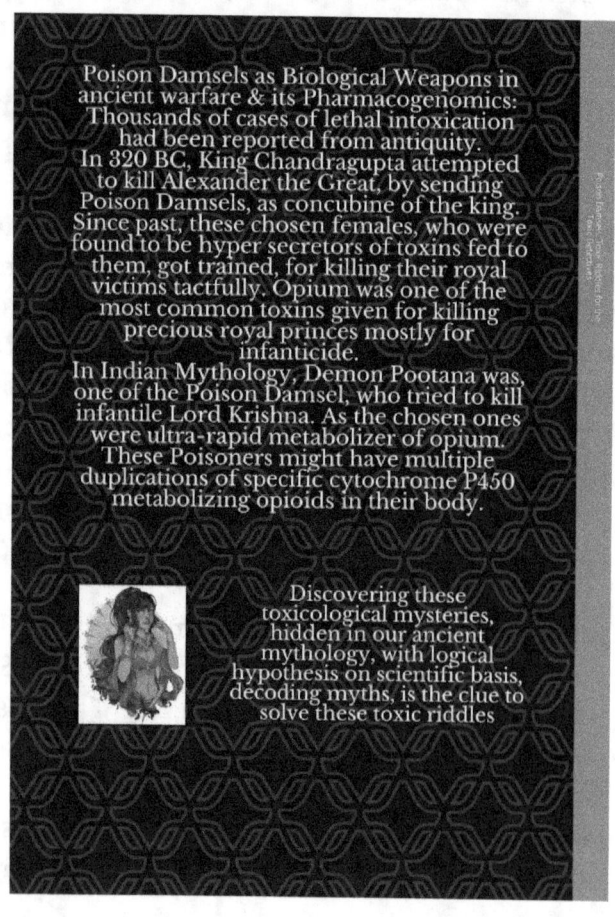

Poison Damsels as Biological Weapons in ancient warfare & its Pharmacogenomics: Thousands of cases of lethal intoxication had been reported from antiquity.
In 320 BC, King Chandragupta attempted to kill Alexander the Great, by sending Poison Damsels, as concubine of the king. Since past, these chosen females, who were found to be hyper secretors of toxins fed to them, got trained, for killing their royal victims tactfully. Opium was one of the most common toxins given for killing precious royal princes mostly for infanticide.
In Indian Mythology, Demon Pootana was, one of the Poison Damsel, who tried to kill infantile Lord Krishna. As the chosen ones were ultra-rapid metabolizer of opium. These Poisoners might have multiple duplications of specific cytochrome P450 metabolizing opioids in their body.

Discovering these toxicological mysteries, hidden in our ancient mythology, with logical hypothesis on scientific basis, decoding myths, is the clue to solve these toxic riddles